Dee

confirmation -
UWO
Oct 78'
may you live long!
Ron

HOW TO LIVE WITH YOUR HIGH BLOOD PRESSURE

HOW TO LIVE WITH YOUR HIGH BLOOD PRESSURE

WILLIAM A. BRAMS, M.D.

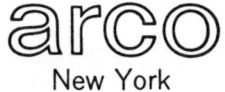
New York

Published by Arco Publishing Company, Inc.
219 Park Avenue South, New York, N.Y. 10003

Copyright © 1956, 1973 by William A. Brams
All rights reserved

Library of Congress Catalog Card Number 72-85751
ISBN 0-668-02695-2

Printed in the United States of America

Figures 7, 8, 9, and 10 adapted from Public Health Service Publication No. 1409 by courtesy of U.S. Department of Health, Education and Welfare

Contents

Preface to the Second Edition	1
Preface to the First Edition, 1956	4
1. The Problem of High Blood Pressure	7
2. High Blood Pressure: A Disease by Itself or a Symptom of a Disease	13
3. Pressure Makes Your Blood Circulate	18
4. Two Types of High Blood Pressure: Their Symptoms	23
5. Who Gets High Blood Pressure?	34
6. Finding a Doctor	44
7. What the Doctor Can Do for You	47
8. How the Doctor Examines You and Why	56
9. What You Can Do for Yourself	75
10. Complications of Essential High Blood Pressure	94
11. Secondary Hypertension: Symptom of Underlying Ailment	107
12. Living with High Blood Pressure: Rules for the Hypertensive	125
13. The Promise of Science	130
Appendix I: Charts Showing Desirable Weights	133
Appendix II: Reducing Diets	135
Appendix III: Agencies of Rehabilitation and Vocational Placement	139
Index	143

HOW TO LIVE WITH YOUR HIGH BLOOD PRESSURE

Preface to the Second Edition

Remarkable advances have been made in modern times in our conception and treatment of high blood pressure, its complications, and what patients can do to help themselves.

The aim of this updated and revised edition is to present a total picture, to disseminate information and understanding through fairly detailed explanations without being overly technical nor yet too general for the curious reader who is interested in hypertension. Among the new developments are many that have not been adequately interpreted to the 20,000,000 among the laity who are hypertensive. Consequently, their families and friends may find this book useful in helping the hypertensive member. Such whole information is not likely to reach non-professional people; they may read piecemeal reports in the newspapers or magazine articles which may or may not be authoritative, and cannot be sufficiently detailed.

Among the many developments, one of the most startling has been the treatment of kidney ailments. Who would have thought it possible to drain out your blood, remove toxic substances from it, and return it cleansed to your body should your kidneys no longer be able to perform this task? In this way, someone whose kidneys do not function properly is made comfortable, and life is prolonged. Yet, today, this is being done when high blood pressure is associated with kidney ailments. This is more fully explained in this book, as is the event of replacing kidneys that have deteriorated beyond repair with the healthy kidneys of close relatives. Results have been highly satisfactory when a gift kidney is available from a suitable donor. The patient can then expect to live almost a normal life.

Most hypertensive patients will never require such astonishing treatment. For most, medical treatment suffices when it is conscientious, standardized and simplified. Medicines now in use were unheard of not too long ago; they do their job well under the supervision of your doctor and your cooperation with him. Troublesome side effects are few, and effectiveness is not lost after prolonged use. Various combinations of certain approved medicines provide additional beneficial effects without increasing any unwanted side effects of each component. Reputable pharmaceutical companies continue their research for better and better medication.

Evidence has been accumulating that sustained treatment is necessary as soon as a rise in blood pressure is detected. The earlier it is detected, the better, for early treatment defers and often even prevents the development of the usual possible complications: heart disorders, strokes, or kidney impairment. It prevents arteriosclerosis, hardening of the arteries, which is really the responsible factor for those complications *but the development of arteriosclerosis is affected by hypertension. Hypertension predisposes to arteriosclerosis.* Hypertension brought and maintained under control may prevent arteriosclerosis. Other dependent factors dovetail and influence the development of arteriosclerosis; you may read about them in this book.

If you are a hypertensive person, you no longer need to look forward with apprehension to an existence of a saltless, tasteless, unappetizing diet for the rest of your life. But you must be under supervised care; so many influences come to bear on the problem. You cannot diagnose yourself; you cannot treat yourself. Paid advertising spokesmen cannot diagnose you nor treat you. Only your doctor can.

PREFACE TO THE SECOND EDITION

My gratitude to Mrs. Marianne Van Wien, who typed an earlier version of the manuscript.

My willing thankful appreciation goes out to Dr. Morris Fishbein for his helpful direction, and with it, my profound thank-you to Miss Ethel H. Davis for editing the second edition and contributing many helpful suggestions.

An acknowledgment is in order to Mr. Matthew H. Spear, program management officer, Division of Kidney Disease Control, Department of Health, Education and Welfare, for permission to adapt illustrations (Figures 7, 8, 9, and 10) from the Public Health Service publication, number 1409.

Readers, good health and good care to all!

William A. Brams, M.D.
November 14, 1971

Preface to the First Edition, 1956

There are about fifteen million people in the United States whose blood pressure is higher than normal. Although no adequate statistical surveys on low blood pressure are available, its frequency is probably also great.

Naturally, a condition which is so prevalent becomes a matter of great concern to the general public.

The medical profession is informed quickly about new developments in this and other fields of medicine by reading professional journals and by attendance at medical meetings. These channels of information, however, are usually not available to the lay public. The nonprofessional person may thus harbor ideas and conceptions about blood pressure which have long been modified or discarded.

The author feels that it is incumbent upon the medical profession to disseminate the latest views on blood pressure among those who are interested in this subject. Much fear and unwarranted anxiety will thus be avoided and the patient will be enabled to face his problems with better understanding.

The attending physician is, of course, best suited to spread the newer knowledge among his patients. He is not only well-informed, but he also knows his patient intimately and understands his personality pattern, background and problems. There are occasions, however, when lack of time or opportunity prevents a full discussion of blood pressure with every one of his patients and the patient's relatives or friends. A supplementary source of information can then serve a useful purpose.

PREFACE TO THE FIRST EDITION, 1956

In the preparation of this volume, written in simple, non-technical language, the author has kept in mind the following objectives:

a) To place before the lay reader the known facts about blood pressure in its various phases;

b) To evaluate the practical aspects of the more recent developments in the light of seasoned experience and ripe judgment;

c) To outline a more accurate picture of high and low blood pressure in the light of recent achievements rather than in the dark misconceptions of the past.

It will be an agreeable surprise to learn that hypertension—high blood pressure—is very often much more benign than was supposed formerly. It is now known that hypertension frequently produces neither symptoms nor disability for many years and that patients often live out a normal life span in comfort and without undue restriction of normal activities.

The newer knowledge about hypotension—low blood pressure—is even more encouraging. It is now known that the ordinary form of low blood pressure is neither a form of illness nor a sign of impending ill-health. On the contrary, statistical studies indicate that such patients often outlive those who have normal blood pressure.

A very interesting fact which has come to light recently is that many of the symptoms which are encountered in hypertension or in hypotension are due, not to elevation or depression of the blood pressure level, but to accompanying fear, emotional tension, and other character traits of the patient.

Arteries, which bear so much of the brunt of hypertension, are, in fact, very sturdy structures. For example, it has been found that the relatively thin-walled arteries in the brain can withstand internal pressures of from 1,500 to 3,000 millimeters of mercury and more. Such pressures are more than ten to twenty times the normal blood pressure and are many times greater than are found in the most severe forms of hypertension. *We learn from this that it is not the degree of the blood pressure which induces complications. It is the condition of the arteries which determines whether a given patient will remain in good health, despite hypertension.*

These newer concepts, and many others, have revised our ideas radically in recent years. Scientists in many research centers are still studying various aspects of blood pressure. Treatment is not being neglected. In fact, new methods are tested frequently and much progress has been made in the past few years. Although the perfect treatment for all types of hypertension has not yet been found, the search continues and it is not too much to hope that an ideal form of management will soon be available.

The author is particularly grateful to Mrs. Helen MacGill Hughes for many valuable contributions to the text and for adapting the manuscript to the needs of lay readers. Acknowledgment is also made to Dr. Morris Fishbein for his valuable suggestions. The illustrations are by Hertha Furth. Mrs. Arlene Kahn and Miss Connie Ballin, my secretaries, typed the manuscript. Messrs. J. B. Lippincott Company, the publishers, have been very patient and cooperative. Lastly but certainly not least, I owe a debt to my patients, colleagues and students, which, I feel, can never be repaid in full.

William A. Brams, M.D.

Chapter 1

The Problem of High Blood Pressure

You would not be reading this book unless you or someone you know have high blood pressure. I must assume that that is so, and reassure you at once, dear Reader (as old-fashioned novels used to address their readers), that your outlook today is far more favorable than formerly. We doctors can do more for you than ever before to prevent the complications of neglected high blood pressure, and to help you enjoy a long and useful life. We have new understanding about what detrimental conditions may be going on in your body, and we have medicines to control them. In many instances, we do not know why people get high blood pressure; consequently, we do not always know how to prevent it. But in general, help is available, not only by supervised medication of proved value in reducing high blood pressure, but also by certain procedures effective in overcoming possible complications. Not long ago those procedures would have seemed as unimaginable as space travel, now they are all realities.

With each year, we come closer to the full knowledge that we need about the nature of the two types of high blood pressure (for there is more than one type), and how to deal successfully with their effects. In the meantime, Medicine knows enough, so that with care, life may proceed normally provided you follow your doctor's instructions. No, you cannot forget about it; you cannot defy the warnings. Let me give you an example:

"Doctor, please come at once—my husband—he is very sick." The agitated voice over the phone belonged to Mrs. Steele, who was usually calm. She was the wife of a friend of many years. I left for their home immediately. Mr. Steele was propped up on three pillows in a sitting position. His breathing was labored and rapid. I could hear a distinct wheeze each time that he exhaled. He tried to speak but was too out of breath. Mrs. Steele laid a gentle hand on his shoulder. "Relax, John, let me tell the doctor what happened." It was a familiar story to doctors.

Mr. Steele had been working too hard for several months. He had remained at his office for long hours after others had left. Tax time was approaching, a strike was threatening, and needed merchandise had not arrived.

On examination, I heard rattling noises in the patient's chest, indicating severe congestion of the lungs. The heart action was irregular and rapid. The blood pressure was far too high. I gave Mr. Steele an injection to quiet his breathing and to allay his anxiety. I gave him a diuretic pill to increase the output of unwanted body fluid by way of the urine, which, as it did so, would drain the congestion from his lungs while lowering his blood pressure. I then suggested that he be taken to a hospital by ambulance for further treatment. At the hospital the patient received medicine to strengthen his heart and slow its beat; oxygen and other measures brought improvement within several hours. The immediate danger had been overcome. Now my efforts were directed to the basic, the underlying condition: the *high blood pressure*, also called *hypertension*.

High Blood Pressure and Modern Civilization

It is widely believed that high blood pressure is the price of our manner of living amidst our rushed high-geared civilized society. Does this account for the 20 million people in the United States alone who have high blood pressure? Although we are without supporting evidence in this assumption, we cannot deny that the way of modern life may contribute to the development of high blood pressure. By contrast, Chinese in China and Negroes in Africa who live in primitive style seldom have it; whereas it prevails among blacks in New York and Chicago in severer forms than among the white people in those cities and other metropolitan areas. This facet will be taken up again in comments on race.

Your Blood Pressure and Your Daily Experiences

The blood pressure of healthy persons varies with their time of life and, to some extent, with the time of day. Your blood pressure may rise after eating or after exercise, even if the exercise is only a leisurely walk. It may rise when you are tense or nervous or angry. Even the act of measuring a patient's blood pressure, although it entails not the slightest discomfort, may cause the pressure to rise. If the physician talks to the patient for a minute or two until he is more at ease, and then takes the pressure, the second reading will be lower.

Moderate cold elevates the blood pressure; intense cold lowers the blood pressure. Many of you will remember the case of the "Frozen Woman" of Chicago, which showed us that the human body still knows how to hibernate, and in extreme cold can live at a level so low that blood pressure almost disappears. On a night when it was 16° F. below zero, a drunken woman staggered into an alley and fell asleep on the ground. Hours later, when she was found, she was taken to a hospital. The doctors could hardly believe the thermometer when they took her temperature. Instead of the normal 98.6° F., it was 64.4°, the lowest ever known in a living person. Her heart was beating from 12 to 20 beats a minute instead of the normal 70 or 80, and her blood pressure was so reduced that the instruments could not measure it. She lived. As she warmed up, her blood pressure climbed back to normal levels. However, I cannot recommend her method for reducing blood pressure, she paid dearly for the experience with nine frozen fingers and two frozen legs, all of which had to be amputated. The Frozen Woman is a startling demonstration of Nature's provision that the blood pressure shall rise or fall for your body's protection, in response to environment or the experience of the moment. This will be clearer to you as the mechanisms are explained.

Low Blood Pressure (Hypotension)

You have just read that the Frozen Woman's blood pressure was so low that it could not be measured. Although the emphasis in this book is on high blood pressure, perhaps we should at this point explain low blood pressure or hypotension. There is no precise boundary between normal and what may be called low blood pressure in an adult. The standards are arbitrary, adopted for convenience; they may be changed at any future time as new information comes to light.

We recognize three types of *hypotension*: *Primary* or *essential* (not to be confused with *essential hypertension* explained later, page 13), *secondary*, and *postural*. In primary hypotension the cause is unknown. In secondary an underlying recognizable cause is the reason for low blood pressure. In postural, the third type, a less than normal lowering of pressure takes place when a person assumes an upright position.

Primary hypotension occurs in about 3% of the white population in the United States. Just as essential *hypertension* runs in families, so does essential or primary *hypotension*. We do not know why either is familial. Primary hypotension is not an actual illness, and it does not carry a risk of complications as hypertension does.

Hypotensive patients are generally frail young adults, often nervous young women with unstable emotional makeup. Symptoms are never specific; however, the hypotensive person tires easily, often feeling worse fatigue on arising in the morning but recovering later in the day. Weakness and irritability, depression and lack of stamina are probably typical of the patient's personality rather than the result of the low blood pressure.

The condition does not require special treatment other than repeated reassurance and some homemade psychotherapy. It is useful to point out that many with primary (or essential) hypotension live longer than those with normal blood pressure. You see, if you happen to have this type of blood pressure, although you may not have a lot of pep, you will probably live longer than others.

In secondary hypotension, the low blood pressure may set in if you are severely anemic or if you have a longstanding infectious disease. It may also be caused when loss of blood and shock induce the low level, as in battle or traffic injuries in which case the pressure returns to normal or near normal as soon as transfusions and other emergency measures take hold. Other possible causes are certain glandular conditions, nutritional deficiencies, and other bodily deficiencies. In all such cases, the blood pressure may be expected to rise to satisfactory levels when the underlying condition has been corrected.

Postural hypotension takes place when the person assumes an upright position. This type of hypotension is likely in debilitated or elderly people or in those who have been confined to bed for long periods. It may also happen after standing immobile in one spot for some time, especially when emotions are tense. I have seen graduation exercises at the United States Naval Academy at which the cadets (healthy young men) stand motionless in formation so long that after a while, one after another blacks out and falls to the ground. All recover shortly, however, and return to receive their commissions as officers.

I once read an interesting report about women fainting while sightseeing from a bus. The women had sat for hours and hours with their legs down and without moving. All had large varicose veins in their legs in which blood had collected, while other parts of their bodies, including the brain, were deprived of a normal blood supply.

The symptoms of postural hypotension are like those of the secondary form except that they appear when the upright position is assumed perhaps suddenly, or is maintained too long. Recovery follows shortly after lying down. Women find a snug-fitting support garment and support stockings helpful.

On long sightseeing trips, it is advisable to take advantage of all stops by leaving the bus and walking about even if sightseeing has lost its attraction or the tourist feels too tired for museums, monuments and churches.

Chapter 2

High Blood Pressure: A Disease by Itself or a Symptom of a Disease

High Blood Pressure May Be a Disease by Itself or It May Be a Symptom of Another Disease

Your wife may have high blood pressure during pregnancy. Your neighbor may have it in connection with a kidney disorder. Your mother may have experienced it during the menopause (change of life). The man at the next desk may have told you about the high blood pressure he had had when worried while he was out of a job. In all such cases, the high blood pressure is a symptom, the result of some underlying ailment or circumstance. Certain tumors, some glandular disorders, and narrowings in the *aorta* (the main artery from which the whole arterial system proceeds) may cause the blood pressure to rise too high. Other diseases or congenital defects also do this to the pressure, so that the high blood pressure is a *symptom* of those disorders, just as fever or headaches may be symptoms of some disturbance and vanish when the underlying ailment is cured.

In another kind of high blood pressure, which seems to run in families, the condition of the pressure in itself is the only thing wrong; apparently, it is *not* a symptom of something else at all. That type is by far the most frequent form of high blood pressure, called *essential high blood pressure* because the word *essential* means that the high blood pressure is the essence of the trouble, not a symptom of something else. This is the common kind of high blood pressure and therefore receives the most attention in this book, especially because if neglected, it can have consequences.

What Is Normal Blood Pressure?

Your normal blood pressure rises and falls even when you are in the best of health. Even the normal high point and the normal low point for you may not be the same as for your parents or for your children or for your neighbors. If you are like many of my patients, you are too impressed with the numbers that tell how high your blood pressure is. Perhaps you have friends who have the same condition and whenever you meet you compare the scores and frighten yourselves into higher pressures as you talk. You should understand that the numbers by themselves have little meaning. Some people with a blood pressure higher than yours lead normal lives and die at a ripe old age in traffic accidents —not from high blood pressure. Others, whose pressure is normal, are almost invalided, not from pressure but from worry. What, then, is a *normal* blood pressure?

By now, we physicians have measured the blood pressure of thousands and thousands of patients and have learned that no single figure is the *right* blood pressure. Instead, we have adopted an *average range* which we use as a normal reference point. In other words, *any figure within that range* may be considered normal for a particular patient. We do know of healthy people whose blood pressure is above that top limit but we may still consider them in good health. In an experiment at one of the universities, physicians examined 742 presumably healthy students, all young men; about 75 of them had blood pressures higher than the so-called normal range. Apparently it was not too high for those 75.

You may have noticed that your blood pressure is recorded in two figures, one above the other, like a fraction. When we speak of pressure of, say 150, we are telling just half the story. Each time your heart pumps, or gives a "beat," it contracts, squeezing the blood out of its *chambers* and into the *aorta*, that large artery where your body's circulation system begins. (See page 19.) The top figure of the fraction showing your blood pressure is the pressure at the moment when your heart is contracting and thrusting your blood forward into your arteries. This is your *systolic pressure*. The bottom figure of the fraction, always lower, is the pressure when your heart is relaxing between beats. That is known as the *diastolic pressure*.

In a grown person the pressure with which your heart drives blood into the arteries will vary according to age, about which more is said a bit later. But in general, we speak of the normal range of systolic pressure as being between 100 and 145, and the normal range between beats, the diastolic pressure, as being from 70 to 95. These are arbitrary figures, but are universally accepted *ranges* of normal blood pressure in human adults.

Let me tell you that you cause yourself needless worry if you insist on trying to find out the score when your blood pressure is being measured. The figures must be interpreted in the light of medical experience; your physician takes many other factors into consideration. What follows is an example of how meaningless the figures by themselves can be:

A hard-driving, 35-year-old industrialist consulted me because of high blood pressure. His condition was first detected during a routine physical examination when he was 16 years old. It was a surprise to him because he had felt well, even when working hard on his father's farm. Since then, he had undergone several thorough examinations, including electrocardiograms, kidney studies, and numerous other tests, but an underlying cause had not been disclosed. The only symptoms he had through the years were occasional headaches or nervousness when confronted by some serious business problem or when he was upset by an emotional experience. The patient had always been a compulsive eater. He had to eat, hungry or not.

At first, the blood pressure reached high levels periodically with normal intervals lasting several weeks. During the previous 9 years, however, the blood pressure remained high constantly. The patient had had no difficulties while playing football on the first team at college. Afterward he had worked hard and traveled a great deal in connection with his occupation. Because he knew that high blood pressure was undesirable, and that his overeating was a factor (on at least one occasion he had consumed a meal containing 11 large heavily salted perch prepared in oil, accompanied by many side dishes), he tried a rice diet. He could not tolerate the rice diet longer than a few weeks, although his weight was reduced somewhat and so was his pressure.

On my initial examination, the patient weighed 305 pounds and his systolic blood pressure (see page 15) was 230 and his diastolic as high as 135. I prescribed a well balanced reducing diet designed to cause weight reduction of 1 to 2 pounds a week, medicines to reduce the blood pressure gradually, and tranquilizers to be taken as needed. He took his medicines as instructed, but his compulsions to eat prevented his adhering to the prescribed diet. His compulsions to eat were so strong that he actually went into a panic, became weak and dizzy when his weight dropped 3 pounds in a week. Reassurances and coaxing brought his weight down a little, fluctuating between 280 and 300 pounds. His blood pressure remained virtually unchanged. At no time did the patient feel it necessary to rest or slow his pace; still, his physical condition was not deteriorating.

The patient's total known duration of high blood pressure for 45 years shows that high blood pressure alone can be tolerated without disability, provided complications do not result. But how can one be sure that complications will not result? On the surface, that patient was so obese and his pressure was so high that complications might certainly have been expected. His was doubtless an exceptional case in escaping complications; but obviously, although he was not happy with his condition, he managed to live with only high blood pressure and his obesity as abnormalities. In most cases they would have been sufficient to bring about more serious consequences. The example should not justify your neglecting hypertension and overweight, if you are hypertensive and overweight.

CHAPTER 3

Pressure Makes Your Blood Circulate

Reader, you may, if you wish, skip this chapter; however, if you do not know how your blood circulates and are curious about it, here is a simple explanation, a little lesson.

The heart and all the blood vessels form a closed circuit in which the heart acts as a powerful pump and the vessels conduct blood to and from all parts of the body. When the smaller vessels behind the *arteries* (the *arterioles*) become contracted, the arteries behind the arterioles still keep on receiving blood from the pumping heart. The pressure builds up in the arteries, and *the blood pressure rises*. Now, if you want more details about this fascinating system of circulation, read on.

Dissolved in the blood are the oxygen and other nutrient substances needed to keep your cells alive throughout the body; it is the blood that carries the oxygen and nutrition everywhere along the miles and miles of vessels in the body. On its return trip, the blood also picks up the waste products, such as carbon dioxide, to be extruded from the body by the kidneys, bowels, the glands of perspiration, the lungs.

You stand erect, with your head 5 feet or 6 feet from the ground, yet the blood flows uphill all the way to your head. It can do this because the heart is a muscle, a powerful muscle, which forces the blood upward, just as an old-fashioned pump raises water from the well. To keep anywhere from 5 quarts to 7 quarts of blood endlessly circulating in the closed system requires force, or pressure. A large person needs more blood; a small person needs less blood.

Because the heart during its beats rests as often as it works, it can carry on without ceasing, beating 100,800 times each day of your life. (This is a good place to reflect that the heart can teach you something: You will last longer, too, if you rest frequently.) That main artery called the *aorta* carries blood out—away from the heart. In the aorta, the pressure is highest because it receives the full force of the impact of the blood as it is ejected by the powerful *left ventricle* of the heart (one of the two lower chambers of the heart). Soon after the point at which the aorta starts, it sends branches into the head, the trunk, the arms and legs; the branches in turn divide again and again, until they finally taper off into the tiny vessels called arterioles (referred to at the beginning of this chapter). These arterioles have an external diameter of about 1/125th of an inch, hardly large enough to see with the naked eye. The arterioles, small as they are, have comparatively thick muscular walls which enable those tiny vessels to act as nozzles for the ends of the whole arterial system. When the muscular layers of the arterioles contract, their channels become narrower, so that the onward flow of blood is hindered. The flow is hindered enough to slow up but not to stop. The heart goes right on pumping blood into the arteries. As a result (this was explained previously), the blood pressure builds up and rises in all arteries behind the constricted arterioles.

That is not all. The arterioles divide into even smaller blood vessels, known as *capillaries*, a word meaning tiny hairs. The capillaries are just wide enough to permit red blood cells to pass through them in single file. Their walls are unbelievably thin. In this way your capillaries expose every single blood cell with its oxygen and nutrition to the tissues of your body. No matter where you cut yourself, you bleed, because this maze of blood vessels reaches absolutely everywhere in order to feed the millions and millions of cells in the body. After the blood passes through the capillaries, the blood begins its return journey to the heart. As already hinted, it is on this part of the circuit that the blood takes on a sort of scavenger's job, carrying off waste by way of the *veins*, which are a continuation of the capillaries.

The blood in the arteries, stored with life-giving oxygen, is bright red; the blood in the veins is dark, bluish red, because it contains so much less oxygen than when it is in the arteries. It also contains the waste products which it is bearing off. If you are light-skinned, you can see the veins, like blue cords, in the back of your hand, especially if you hold the hand down for a while. Even black people, whose veins seem black, in reality have veins with a bluish cast.

The veins join one another again and again, getting bigger each time until finally they unite into two large veins: the *superior* or *upper vena cava*, and the *inferior* or *lower vena cava*. The two large veins empty their blood into the *right auricle*, one of the two upper chambers of the heart. (You have already read about the *left ventricle*, one of the two lower chambers of the heart.) From the right auricle, which may be thought of as a collecting reservoir, the blood flows into the *right ventricle*, a lower chamber. Because of its thick and strong walls, the right ventricle drives the blood into the capillary network of the lungs for refueling with oxygen. The gaseous waste products, which the blood had been collecting on its return journey to the heart, pass into the air spaces of the lungs, from which it is breathed out. Now the blood leaves the lungs to enter the *left auricle* of the heart, the other upper chamber, which acts as a collecting reservoir for the blood that has re-entered the heart from the lungs. From the left auricle the blood then enters the powerful left ventricle which pumps the blood with great force into the aorta. As already described, the aorta blood is pumped to all parts of the body. The cycle completed, it is repeated over and over, so that the blood is circulating through the body every moment of the day and night.

The heart and arteries can also adapt themselves to varying conditions within the body. For example, when we run for a bus, our muscles require more blood, just as the motor of the automobile requires more gasoline when we wish to travel faster. To meet this contingency, the heart beats faster and pumps out more blood per minute, and the arteries open more widely in order that the muscles may receive a larger supply of blood.

When loss of blood is severe, as may happen in an accident, an important redistribution of the reduced amount of blood available in the body takes place. Arteries supplying less important regions of the body become constricted, thus reducing the amount of blood sent to those parts. At the same time, the arteries that deliver blood to vital regions, such as the brain or heart, do not become constricted, so that a larger proportion of the total blood in the body may be diverted to the vital organs, which need the blood most.

All that has been described applies to the circulatory system when all is in order. In contrast to man-made machines, the heart, blood vessels, and blood repair themselves to a remarkable extent when damaged, short of fatally. No one thinks anything of an automobile when left at the garage for the repair of a part; but everyone is dismayed when an organ of the body does not function as it should. An injury to the heart can heal, under appropriate care; a clot plugging an artery or vein can be liquefied and absorbed, and red blood cells can be replaced. Such repairs and replacements happen constantly during our entire lifetime. No factory or machine can equal this record for maintenance and production, for service without a strike or holiday. One day, a time-out for resting to allow repair to take place may become necessary. And medical assistance may have to intervene; even surgical aid may be indicated. Today, these are available. The heart and its system of vessels and circulating blood have incomparable ability for restoration, if they are treated as they deserve. This built-in ability should fill us with wonder and admiration, especially when we think of the endless assaults to this built-in system in the course of a lifetime. Some harmful assaults such as eating, over-working, sometimes dissipations, worrying, stresses, and anger, *may* first show their effect in a constantly maintained rise in blood pressure, a warning that must be heeded.

Wonders are many [in life] *and none is more wonderful than man.*— Sophocles*

*I hope that readers among the Women's Lib movement do not take offense. Women are equally wonderful. Sophocles used the word "man" in the sense of mankind (or womankind); that is, human beings.

CHAPTER 4

Two Types of High Blood Pressure: Their Symptoms

The symptoms of high blood pressure depend on what type of hypertension you have. There are two types: *essential* and *secondary*.

Essential Hypertension: In this type, the cause is not apparent; therefore, we do not yet know exactly what it is. We do know that the blood pressure is higher than it should be. It may be that only the systolic pressure is too high, or both the systolic and diastolic pressures may be too high. Of the two, the diastolic pressure is the more important; but, by no means may we disregard the elevated systolic pressure when it alone is a symptom. Studies have shown that even systolic elevation carries a risk of leading to ultimate complications should it be neglected. This aspect is discussed under *Treatment*.

Secondary Hypertension: Here the high blood pressure is *one of the symptoms of an underlying illness*. The underlying illness can usually be detected, and if it is detected and eradicated, the blood pressure returns to normal or near normal. The symptoms in this type are those of the underlying illness in addition to the rise in blood pressure which cannot be treated without treatment of the basic disorder. Examples of such underlying conditions are discussed separately in Chapter 11.

Symptoms of Essential Hypertension: About one third of patients with essential hypertension are without any symptoms whatever for as long as 10 or 20 years; occasionally, even for longer periods. It may first be detected accidentally in the course of a routine health checkup, examination for employment, for college entrance, for permission to participate in strenuous sports, for life insurance, or for military service, even though you feel perfectly well and are without symptoms. The symptoms in the remaining two thirds of patients are vague and variable. I believe strongly that many times the symptoms are not caused by the elevated blood pressure itself but by the basic ailment.

Headaches are common and they can be severe. They are usually felt at the back or top of the head, awakening the patient early in the morning. Dizziness, fatigue, nervousness, palpitation, weakness, and insomnia may be other symptoms. Who has not had such symptoms with *normal* blood pressure? But the symptoms pass; they are transitory. It is their persistence and increasing intensity that must not be disregarded nor masked by over-the-counter or over the TV "cure-alls." (See also *Warnings on Headaches*, this chapter.)

In the early stages, the rise in blood pressure is often periodic, with long intervals of normal pressure. The blood pressure may rise while studying for a difficult school examination, during excitement, or during a period of hard sustained work. The most frequent precipitating factor at the early stage is emotional upset or a series of such upsets: fear, anger, quarrels, anxiety, and violent feelings of any kind. They are experienced chiefly in the brain and in the body, as the brain sends out messages to alert your various parts and organs to what is going on in it.

Our hair does not stand on end visibly as a scared cat's does nor do we bare our fangs in rage as a snarling dog does. But the sensations are there, and when we get into a bitter argument or suffer a severe shock, the same sort of change takes place in our glands, in our hearts, and in our breathing as happens in animals. Such changes are *preparation* for action: for fight or flight. If we are too controlled and too civilized to use our fists and teeth, our bodies still carry on with the old instinctives and prepare for the fray. Thus, even though it is only a battle of words, our blood pressure rises as the blood courses through our bodies to activate the brain and the limbs that will be called on for extra efforts. In the healthy, that rise in blood pressure is transitory; in the hypertensive it lasts longer. That is why we must avoid worry and prevent violent scenes as much as possible. If you have hypertension, worry and anger make it worse. That stage of periodic high blood pressure may last for many years. Eventually the duration of hypertension becomes longer and longer; the normal intervals become shorter and shorter. Finally, the rise in blood pressure becomes sustained; it remains high without relief or with only minor fluctuations.

It may be somewhat consoling to learn that it is not the height of the blood pressure nor its constancy that determines if or when complications may occur. It is the condition of the arteries that affects this; however, hypertension in some way seems to favor the development of arteriosclerosis. This condition favors the development of blood clots in the channels of the arteries; it weakens the walls of the arteries, causes them to break and hemorrhage. Hypertension seems also to favor the narrowing of the channels, thereby interfering with the flow of blood through the vessels. Thus, complications such as the following occur: heart failure, heart attacks, strokes, kidney disorders, or (when the arteries in the legs are the ones affected) interference with walking.

Warnings on Headaches: The headache is probably all too familiar to you. Of all the complaints that my patients bring me, headaches are the most frequent. Other physicians give the same report, stating that usually more than half of their hypertensive patients have pains in the head. If the headaches are severe enough and frequent enough, they may drive you to see a doctor. It is fortunate that headaches usually come in the early stage of hypertension when the doctor can treat you most effectively. However, we learn from many of our hypertensive patients who are about 45, that they have been having headaches for months or even years. Severe and persistent headaches can make one highly nervous, so that the blood pressure rises still more. That is an important reason to seek help without delay.

The pain may be in the back of the head, as has been said, but it may be in the temples, in the top or sides of the head; most feel pain at the back of the head and neck. Some patients say that it is not a real headache, but a full, tight feeling in the head and scalp. Often the head pains come at the unwelcome hour of dawn, waking you too early and keeping you miserable until the alarm clock goes off and you must get up and face the world. Head pain may be at its worst at breakfast, then wear off as you move about. The known facts regarding the reason for headaches accompanying hypertension are confusing. Anxiety and emotional tension provide a plausible explanation. One notable experiment in England almost persuaded the medical profession that headaches come from worry rather than the high blood pressure itself. Several London doctors studied 200 hypertensive patients, some of whom already knew that they had hypertension; the others did not. To everyone's astonishment, nearly all those who knew that they had hypertension had headaches, but only a small proportion of those who did not know it told of this symptom. Other studies show that many patients began to notice headaches precisely at the time when they were first told that they had hypertension.

The evidence does not all point one way. Often the customary time for the headaches is before being properly awake, presumably at a time when one is not worrying, perhaps not yet even thinking. If worry induces the headaches, then logically they should come later in the day when the cares of the world are crowding in on you. On this point, logic does not seem to help understanding, because typically the headaches are likely to subside later in the day. Medicine is certain of one fact, that is, a connection between headaches and hypertension does exist. Whenever we succeed in bringing down a patient's high blood pressure, whether by medication or change in diet and habits of daily life, headaches almost invariably stop *unless* the headache is caused by another ailment.

Aches and Pains: You may be plagued, as many people are, by pains in other places besides your head. My patients tell of aches across the shoulder blades, in the arms, the legs, the back. Some think that they have arthritis or neuritis. Others notice that they feel worse when tense and nervous and that relief comes when they are relaxed, and from this they conclude that the "trouble" is nerves. But it could also be that blood pressure is at its highest. For the most part those pains also vanish when the blood pressure is brought under control.

Dizziness: Hypertensive patients are likely to be annoyed by uncomfortable sensations of dizziness, as though they were swaying or about to fall in a faint. Actually, they rarely do faint; it is just a feeling that passes off almost at once. Sometimes it takes the form called *vertigo*, a sensation that the world is spinning about you or that you yourself are whirling the way a top spins. Dizziness and vertigo come on suddenly and are fleeting during an abrupt change of position, as in bending over to put one's shoes on or to pick up something from the floor, or in sitting up in bed or turning around. We do not know why dizziness goes along with hypertension. Some authorities are of the opinion that it is due to poor circulation in the ears where the balancing apparatus is located; but that is still just a theory.

Emotional Symptoms: Many young or middle-aged women with high blood pressure have a tendency to tears. They weep; but they do not mean to and do not know why. They may be embarrassed by unaccountable blushing. This is not the usual pink glow, but a deep, blotchy flushing all over the face and neck. With it, according to what many patients tell me, comes a feeling that the heart is racing and pounding. It all passes, and is not serious in itself. Reader, for your own peace of mind, endure it but try to forget it, for it never lasts long. If such symptoms are caused by high blood pressure, after your doctor has brought the blood pressure down to a wholesome level, with your cooperation, the symptoms will disappear.

Tiredness and Wakefulness: You may be one of those luckless persons who wakes up tired or who tires quickly. Although you begin the day energetically, your endurance is limited and your strength seems exhausted by midafternoon. Even your brain seems tired and it is hard to concentrate as well as you used to do. Insomnia may make the situation worse. The sleep that you hope will revive you, "Nature's soft nurse," as Shakespeare called it, will not come. Or, you may drop off to sleep quickly, but wake up at three or four in the morning and after that, no matter how many sheep you count, you cannot sleep. My own theory is that counting sheep or any other game does not have the desired effect; it starts you thinking and one thought leads to another. The secret is to dismiss everything from the mind; you can do nothing about anything at that hour anyway. Above all, do not listen to the siren songs of TV commercials and all the nostrums that they try to entice you to try, to rid you of headaches, pains anywhere, or insomnia. They mask symptoms, so that you delay seeking professional advice. They may be harmless in themselves, but they are also of no use to you in rooting out the cause. You are an individual who deserves individual examination and personalized treatment. The handsome actor or the alluring actress or the paid TV advertiser are all just reading the script written by an advertising agency. It is the modern equivalent of the old medicine man of pioneer days whose bottle cured everything. Those people are not qualified to tell you what is good for you.

Crossness: It is small wonder that with trials by day and night—headaches, fatigue, insomnia—you are not the best company in the world. One might say of the combination of pain and insomnia what Mark Twain said of St. Vitus dance and rheumatism. He nominated them as the two worst things to have at the same time. If your family complains that you are an irritable, impatient, restless worrywart, at least you have your reasons. You may magnify trifles, take a gloomy view of life, and interpret everything about yourself as an ominous symptom. This is an unfortunate habit of mind, for as a rule, things are not as bad as you imagine. Even if they are, if you can do something about them, do; if not, your state of mind only complicates a situation. All that your unfortunate state of mind can do is keep your blood pressure higher longer.

See Your Doctor Now! What He Can Do for You

Your high blood pressure may not be causing you any discomfort yet, or even doing you any great harm *yet*. If you have somehow found out that you have the condition, you would be wise to realize that you have been forewarned and should see your doctor as soon as possible. He will begin systematic measures, under his direction, to correct the disturbance. Emphatically, do not ask advice from amateurs. Do not compare notes with others who say that they have the same trouble. They are not trained to interpret symptoms; different disorders may have the same or similar symptoms. Above all, do not take medicines that a friend or a paid testimonial by a well known person tells you helped him: "So why don't you try it?" The roads to hypertension are many and the ways in which your type of hypertension may differ from another's and should be treated are just as many. The medicines that helped another may be useless or even harmful to you. The man on TV does not know you; he is not licensed to prescribe. The nostrum he peddles may be compared with the magic potion of earlier years purporting to do all things for all people. He is selling quackery in one of the modern forms still with us. In the same way, the many "doctor" programs on TV should be taken with a barrel of salt. They are not for viewing as if they were educational and authentic documentary films. At best what the actors are portraying may not apply to you at all. What is worse, the script writer may have distorted the facts to fit his plot, or he may not have understood the facts in the first place.

Because every one of the symptoms that I have mentioned may or may not be due to hypertension in itself, your doctor's work is sometimes like that of a detective's. He must follow clues and explore possibilities that may apply to you. If anyone close to you has begun to notice any of the symptoms mentioned, urge him to seek medical aid. Because hypertension often runs in families, it is particularly necessary for you to go to your doctor at once if your parents, grandparents, sisters or brothers have or had high blood pressure. Reap the advantage of Nature's signals. The wisdom of regular medical checkups is demonstrated by the frequent accidental awareness of having hypertension brought about through the routine physical examination required of you for some other purpose previously mentioned. It is foolish to put your health last and everything else first. You do not need to feel miserable, struggling to keep going all the while that you are fighting avoidable pain and sleeplessness. "Over the counter" pharmaceuticals will probably only mask the reason for your symptoms. Your doctor can bring those discomforts and others under healthful control. Give him the chance to help you while the chance is good. Do not become an emergency through neglect. Help your doctor help you to a livable measure of comfort and well-being. It takes an expert to interpret and to prescribe. Do not try to be your own doctor and do not delay!

When complications are the first evidence that you have of high blood pressure, it is no longer evidence of hypertension alone. It is evidence that you have had high blood pressure for many years, and waited for the development of complications that requires treatment. For the sake of fuller illustration, I have intentionally picked from my records a severe example of a patient who learned suddenly that his blood pressure was too high.

The Case of the Man Who Was Too Busy

Mr. Bartlett had begun to notice that he got out of breath when climbing stairs. He did not feel well at the end of the day. Even worse, he woke up tired in the morning and had to force himself to do what used to come easily. He thought this was because he was overweight and that if he could lose about 40 pounds, he would feel more energetic. Then he began to have headaches, usually early in the morning. His neck and shoulders hurt him. Finally, he decided that he ought to see his doctor. But he was too busy at the time and kept putting it off; you know how that is.

Mr. Bartlett was a successful business man. But from the way he drove himself, one would think that he was staving off bankruptcy. He worked early and worked late; weekends and holidays meant nothing to him. He was a perfectionist. (Are you?) If he set himself a goal or made a promise, he accomplished it, no matter how inconvenient or at what cost to himself, and others. He had been working especially hard at the factory in connection with an order, and tiring more and more, but the job was to be finished in another week and he kept at it. He had promised himself that when it was finished, he was going to take life easier, and would see the doctor. But he had pushed his luck too long.

One morning he awoke early with the feeling of weights on his chest. Frightened, he struggled to sit up, gasping for breath. He felt strange; gurgling sounds came from his throat and chest but he could not control them. Pink froth dribbled from the corners of his mouth, and he felt sick and confused. Later on, when he tried to recall that morning, he remembered a doctor bending over him and giving him a hypodermic injection. The next thing he knew, he was in the hospital. A rubber mask, like a soldier's gas mask, covered his face and a tank stood beside the bed. This apparatus was there to give him oxygen to relieve the condition in his lungs, although he was too ill at the time to understand it.

Every morning I went to see Mr. Bartlett at the hospital. I talked to him, explaining his illness. I told him his blood pressure was high; overwork, worry, eating too much and sleeping too little had caused too great a load for his body. The heart had been receiving more blood than it could pump out, so that the blood had backed up into his lungs. That accounted for the pressure on his chest, the difficulty in breathing, and the bringing up of blood.

Fortunately, Mr. Bartlett recovered as most such patients do. No amount of good counsel would have induced a man like that to change his habits while there was still time;

but fright forced him to realize that he was really destroying himself with his frenzied pace of working. During his hospital stay, Mr. Bartlett for the first time faced the fact that success in business was not worth it, if the price was his own health. He had had warning signals but had disregarded them. Yet, had he understood them, he might have avoided that brush with death.

CHAPTER 5

Who Gets High Blood Pressure?

Although we do not know the actual cause of essential hypertension, we are well informed about certain conditions favoring its development. Bear in mind that these are not causes, but having those conditions makes a person more *susceptible* to getting high blood pressure. Those predisposing conditions are: heredity, family history, temperament and emotional stability, age, sex, race, obesity and body build.

Heredity is an important factor in making one *susceptible* to the development of essential hypertension. Essential hypertension runs in families. It is not invariable; some with a family history of high blood pressure escape it themselves. Others, without hypertension among their parents and grandparents, can become the first of the line. They may introduce it to some of their descendants. The figures tell the tale:

In one study of many family histories of patients, 3% had hypertension when both parents had *normal* blood pressure. When one parent had it, the rate rose to 28%. If both parents had it, the rate rose to 45%. This is so striking that we see it as a clue to the secret of what causes hypertension in the first place; but the mystery remains unsolved. Your doctor will ask you, though, if any of your near relatives have or had hypertension. It is a routine question put to every patient regardless of the reason for consulting a doctor. If you answer affirmatively, your doctor is immediately alerted. You should also be alerted if you have such a family background, and seek consultation with a doctor even if you are without symptoms. We do not know what the hereditary element is, but the medical profession is studying its patients, case by case, in the hope of discovering why this susceptibility persists from one generation to another in the family line.

Temperament and emotional stability, as predisposing factors, are almost as important as heredity. Everyone has moments of flaring bad temper or gnawing anxiety. Blood pressure rises at such times in all of us; in normal persons, it soon subsides. Doctors have learned to recognize a "hypertensive type," perpetually worried, easily provoked, a perfectionist who drives others because of this trait. His nerves are forever crying havoc, never calm and at peace. The muscles about his mouth, eyes, and forehead show the strain. His tenseness, his unrelaxed manner of sitting, and his nervous speech betray the emotional storms tormenting him.

The strain of a routine insurance or military physical examination provokes an abnormally high jump in blood pressure. The exaggerated behavior of the blood pressure often becomes set in adolescence. We are learning now to predict that a particular apparently tireless high school athlete, or that powerfully built, enduring young soldier, reacting excessively as he does to the stress and strain of daily existence, will almost certainly become hypertensive by the time he is 40 years old. This is more likely if both his parents have or had high blood pressure. The type who becomes boisterous and exhibits outbursts of noisy hilarity on slight occasion is also likely to have high or higher blood pressure with each such episode. May I digress to describe briefly a patient of mine who might be called the "laughing lady"?

Some years ago, I undertook a special study of high

blood pressure among patients who were overweight. One, a jolly stout lady was being tested at five-minute intervals to discover whether her pressure was steady or variable. The systolic readings were between 170 and 180 until I chanced to make her laugh. Immediately her blood pressure rose to 300 and stayed there for 15 minutes. It may even have been higher but that was the top reading of the *sphygmomanometer*, the instrument for measuring the blood pressure. My own blood pressure must have been high at that moment of observing her heightened pressure. My patient realized that I was watching her but saw no reason for my reaction. So she laughed more and more. Nothing happened then except that her face was flushed. Mine must have been ashen. As the joke wore off, the mercury in the sphygmomanometer glided down the tube to the earlier level of a little over 170. Insofar as I could judge, she was none the worse for the incident. We do not all have arteries as evidently durable as hers.

In normal people, passing moods raise the blood pressure temporarily. In persons predisposed to hypertension, or those who already have hypertension, the elevation rises higher and lasts longer.

Regarding *age* and *sex*, hypertension is uncommon up to the age of 20. From then up to the age of about 40, men normally have higher blood pressure than women. That is why it is foolish for husbands and wives to judge their own blood pressure by their partners'. In middle life the differences become less noticeable. After the menopause (change of life or climacteric), women become more susceptible to hypertension than men. For some middle-aged women, high blood pressure is only one of several temporary discomforts. Many are unhappy at this period of their lives, facing the reality that the children are grown and do not need them and that their husbands have meanwhile got into the habit of permitting their business to cut into leisure. Fathers still have their work and perhaps a hobby or sport outlet; mothers, however, find themselves virtually unemployed as homemaker after years of many responsibilities. Unless they have planned ahead for an occupation when the day would come with more freedom to pursue neglected interests (as more women do today than formerly), loneliness, a feeling of being worthless and perhaps unwanted come poorly timed when hot flashes and other physical annoyances or disturbances may occur. It is important to recognize that some diseases happen to coincide with the same period of life in which the menopause falls and may not be a part of that crisis at all.

A prepared attitude and prearranged activities help many women breeze through this biological turn without an emotional upheaval at all, particularly if they have guarded their health and have remained free of illnesses that come or may come to anyone, and if, at the same time, they have readied themselves for a suitable refuge from the loneliness of having children leave home. The blood pressure, however, may rise as incident to the biologic and emotional adjustments necessary when these altered circumstances loom large. Usually it all passes, and with it the hypertension which in most instances happens to develop, not because of the change of life, but as a coincidence at that time.

In both sexes, blood pressure rises moderately with age, the systolic blood pressure more so than the diastolic (see page 15). That in itself is no reason to become upset. Blood pressure rising with accumulating years is natural, so long as the arteries are sound; it, in itself, causes no harm. If you have not had hypertension by the age of 50, it is unlikely that you will ever have it. If you do have it, it must be brought down under control. How can you tell how long the arteries will remain sound in the presence of hypertension?

If you are between 40 and 49 years of age, your blood pressure may be above what would have been considered normal in your youth. This is so for 20 or 30 people in a hundred. Between the ages of 50 and 59, 40 of every 100 people have pressures that would seem high in a young person; between the ages of 60 and 69, 50 in every 100, and between the ages of 70 and 79, 66 in every 100.

A popular notion is that the normal is 100 plus your age; that is not the case. For your own peace of mind, just forget that myth, even though blood pressure does rise often with advancing age. Are you among those people who cannot resist tormenting themselves by their interest in blood pressure levels? Remember that if your blood pressure is significantly higher than what it was when you first took out life insurance (perhaps 25 years or more previously), your fears are entirely in order.

Races or *strains of human beings* are basically alike. Striking visible differences appear only in color of the hair, eyes, and skin, in physique and facial features. We are not so varied as are the strains of dogs, for example. It comes as a surprise, therefore, that less obvious wide differences in susceptibility to illnesses are real.

The Chinese seem lucky to have had some sort of immunity to hypertension while in their native country. We do not yet know whether this still holds under their political regime of the last twenty-five years. In that respect other peoples are equally lucky while they remain in their homelands: the native Australians, Filipinos, Mexicans, Cubans (or at least, they were), Puerto Ricans, the American Indians, and non-urban Negroes in Africa whose susceptibility rises in the great cities of the United States. Blacks have hypertension at an earlier age than their white fellow citizens in the United States. Twice as many hypertensive persons were found among the black factory workers of a Cincinnati industry as compared with the same number of white employees. In South Africa the city-bred Bantu is an exception to the apparent rule that Africans are immune. Perhaps that condition is offset by the environment.

An interesting and rather puzzling result of a research project among the Jewish hypertensive population in New York City disclosed that the well-to-do seem about as susceptible as the well-to-do non-Jewish population. But the poor among them are proportionately oftener hypertensive than the poor among non-Jews. Moreover, Jewish New Yorkers, although they commonly have essential hypertension, are relatively free of the symptomatic high blood pressure accompanying kidney disease. When we finally discover the cause of essential hypertension, it will be fascinating to see how the newer knowledge will make sense of such bewildering circumstances.

The Michigan Heart Association released a report in October, 1971, saying that the color and shade of your skin and where you live could determine how likely you are to have high blood pressure. That report agreed that on a percentage basis more blacks have high blood pressure than whites, according to a 1968-1969 survey of 1000 persons. The report was entitled "Socio-Ecological Stress and Black-White Blood Pressure in Detroit." It showed also that light-skinned white women have a greater tendency to high blood pressure than dark-skinned white women.

Some argue that the stress and insecurity of poverty-stricken city black people cause high blood pressure among them. Perhaps so; but then why do the urban well-to-do blacks have it (and some are well-to-do or moderately comfortable) as much as white well-to-do business and professional men? By their own accounts, their trials are worse than Job's: income taxes, incompetent office help, deals that fall through, unloving wives, foolish and ungrateful children, and a hundred other harassments. They will tell you how they envy barefoot, carefree, small town Tom Sawyers and wish they could return to the old days of their boyhood and the simple life of their forebears. That simple life is a fairy tale. We may be pushed and rushed and overworked; but who was more overworked than our pioneer ancestors on the frontier whose lives were grim and grief-ridden? And can the lives of those who lived in slavery be envied by their descendants today even though their conditions varied with their "masters"? Today illnesses that have lost their terror (except in a few still underdeveloped areas of the world) because they are so rare were then rife: cholera, small pox, malaria, typhoid fever, diphtheria, pneumonia, appendicitis, to mention only a few of yesterday's causes of death. Often there was not a doctor anywhere within consoling distance, although had he been at hand his help would have been doubtful, and personally frustrating. If anxiety and tension do it, our forefathers should have had more high blood pressure than we have. Perhaps they did; we will never know. Instruments with which to measure blood pressure had not been invented.

The death-dealing diseases already mentioned, together with tuberculosis, the infections, and the risks of operations have been largely conquered by new concepts of sanitatation and "the miracle drugs," so called by the newspapers. There are penicillin and other antibiotics. Millions now living would have lost their chances of a normal life span, which is normally longer today than in former times. Because the diseases of infancy and childhood are prevented by vaccine injections and birth defects are surgically correctible, more babies now live into maturity than ever before. So we survive the diseases of childhood, the infections, the widespread epidemics but live long enough to have arthritis, certain types of cancer, heart disorders, hardening of the arteries, and high blood pressure. If these are increasing, it is because more people live to middle life and old age.

Is High Blood Pressure Actually Commoner Today?

Today's baby can expect an average life span of about 71 years. This means that some live many years longer, although others may die sooner. The average length of life expectancy in 1900 was only 50 years. The number of Americans who are over 65 is more than four times what it was 50 years ago. Certainly, *if* we have more high blood pressure than our forebears, we can be sure that one reason is our longer life span. But some of the increase may be more apparent than real. Today, doctors recognize abnormal blood pressure. Formerly, high blood pressure was not recognized, because doctors did not know it; they did not look for it; they did not have the instrument (the sphygmomanometer) by which to measure the blood pressure.

There is no reason at all to suppose that hypertension is a new disease. The Egyptians of ancient times had diseases still common today. King Merneptah who was Pharaoh in Egypt at the time of the Hebrew exodus, about 3300 years ago, had hardening of the arteries (arteriosclerosis) in exactly the form familiar to us today. We know this because small pieces of aorta (the main artery from which the whole circulatory system proceeds, described in Chapter 3) taken from his mummy revealed this when examined under a microscope.

In conclusion, we cannot be certain that high blood pressure has as much to do with the pace of modern life as is often supposed. To the extent that medical science has reduced the toll of many other diseases and keeps us alive, in possible comfort, to old age, the increasing high blood pressure may be considered the fly in the ointment of our longer lives, unless accidents or wars get to us first.

Excessive weight and body build appear to affect susceptibility to high blood pressure. It is generally believed that essential hypertension is more common among the following: the obese, especially if they are short, short-necked, and of stocky build, and the hyper-reactors who over-react to circumstances, and exaggerate their responses.

Statistics of life insurance companies covering many, many thousands of men and women, have provided excellent reports connecting overweight with hypertension. Physicians have no doubt that if you are overweight, you are inviting high blood pressure. At the Mayo Clinic, a study of 2,042 patients, aged 15 years and over, showed that with increasing weight the blood pressure rose, as if it were climbing steps. We do not yet understand this relationship. Whatever the basis, we know that losing weight is an absolute necessity for almost all hypertensive persons if complications are to be prevented. The case cited on page 15 was an exception of a man who managed to live without complications despite his compulsive eating and high blood pressure. I would not advise trying to duplicate his luck. The rule was unmistakably demonstrated during and after World War II by the half-starved population of occupied countries who with little food, little fat, had little hypertension. They had other ailments, a great deal of tension, anxiety, worry, and hurts.

How High Can Blood Pressure Go?

As I have said before, the height of blood pressure, in itself, signifies nothing, provided that your arteries endure that rise. Arteries are like an automobile tire filled with air; or like a garden hose filled with water. Their walls are pushed outward when they are filled; as long as they are sound, they can stand considerable pressure. Anatomists have learned from examining unclaimed bodies of young and healthy people who died violent deaths, that the walls of human arteries can stand a pressure of about 3,000 before they will break. If, however, the wall of a tire, a hose or an artery is weakened, it will not stand up so well when the pressure is raised. In normal living, no one's arteries are subjected to a pressure of 3,000. The highest reading I have ever encountered in my practice was about 300, which is as high as the usual instrument will measure.

CHAPTER 6

FINDING A DOCTOR

Let us suppose that you have noticed some of the disturbing symptoms or warnings that I have been describing, and that the headaches, in particular, have become more than you can stand. At last you face the reality that you must see a doctor. But suppose you do not have your own doctor, a common predicament. You may have moved to a new town, or your doctor may have moved away, gone into the Army, or died. How can you find a doctor when you need one? You might ask your former doctor, if he is available, to suggest someone to take his place. If you are moving to another city, he may look up the list of the members of that city's medical society, in the directory of licensed physicians, and choose one for you whose medical training and affiliations sound promising. He may even know the physician personally, or he may ask one of his colleagues whether he knows one of the local physicians personally. The best way to get a reliable doctor is to start with a doctor you already know. An alternative is to consult a friend in the new city whose judgment you trust, and who has lived in the city some time.

If you are a complete stranger and have no one to advise you, then telephone the local hospital. If there is a local medical school, telephone the dean; tell him that you need medical care, and ask him to suggest a physician. Doctors and hospitals usually like to name several possibilities and let you do the choosing. You can be sure that anyone whose name comes to you in this way is reliable. The medical society of a large city may have a doctor referral service. Do not hesitate to ask for this sort of help. Doctors understand your need and are accustomed to such inquiries and they stand ready to see that you do not fall into unscrupulous hands. Quacks are still around despite all the vigilance and efforts to unmask them, and they thrive on the uncautious and the gullible applicant.

Never go to a doctor through some casual connection. Never ask a taxi driver, a redcap or a policeman. They may all be experts at their own business, but not in medicine. They may give you a name that they have seen painted on a window, recall one that they once heard mentioned by a passenger, or may have read in the newspapers. It is possible that they may even be unscrupulous "feeders," for a price sending people to an impostor, a charlatan, a quack, or an incompetent who gets by with such dishonesty. Your body is the only one you have; it is far too important for offhand disposition. Guard it and be on guard when entrusting its care to anyone.

Now let us suppose that you have found a doctor, phoned for an appointment, and have gone to his office. Let us go over his steps one by one in order. As you sit beside his desk, he begins the interesting and sometimes far from simple task of deciding what is wrong with you. Hypertension is not like an obvious wound or a fracture. To the skilled physician, it may be clear immediately that you are not in good health; nevertheless, he does not jump to conclusions. He knows that several possibilities must be considered, because the symptoms of high blood pressure are also symptoms of a number of other disturbances. It is important that you, too, be aware of this and not indulge in self-diagnosis. The doctor watches for clues, follows one for a while, may discard it eventually in favor of a second clue. He continues in this way, drawing on his knowledge and experience, and on laboratory tests until he reaches a likely explanation for your symptoms. This procedure is called *differential diagnosis*. The ultimate or established diagnosis depends on differentiating, and weighing of facts about one likely disorder against others, until the doctor can pinpoint the diagnosis that fits all the facts of your story.

CHAPTER 7

WHAT THE DOCTOR CAN DO FOR YOU

You and the doctor constitute a team; your goal is to win back your good health. This can best be done by cooperation and trust in each other. You must have confidence in your doctor and he must feel assured that you will listen to his advice. You can be at ease that he is trying his best and that he is using the newest, most effective medicines known. After investigations of the effect of certain medications on the market have been made in the laboratory and on human volunteers, your doctor believes with the poet Alexander Pope: "Be not the first by whom the new is tried nor yet the last to lay the old aside." He watches the published reports of reliable physicians and investigators and compares results with his colleagues to make sure that a medication is worth prescribing. Your doctor considers the medicines that may be most suitable for *you*, by appraising your personality, your environment, your needs and how you go about meeting those needs. This information is indispensable to his judgment regarding your conscientiousness in following his instructions.

Specialists who treat patients for high blood pressure observe that some patients fail to improve despite adequate treatment; questioning often discloses that those patients discontinue taking the prescribed medicine, because of indifference or because they think the medicine is not working fast enough.

It has always seemed to me that a patient is likelier to

adhere to instructions if he knows what his doctor is doing. You are entitled to know what medicines you are receiving, what effects they produce, and even why a particular dose is recommended. By providing the patient with enough information, a patient feels that he is indeed a member of the therapeutic team and then he is likely to cooperate. I believe that such teamwork is better than merely writing a prescription and issuing orders on what a patient must or must not do. Most patients can be handled in this manner. However, a great deal depends on the patient's intelligence.

You may well ask whether treatment of high blood pressure today is more effective than it was formerly. Your doctor is certainly better qualified today than a doctor was a scant 25 years ago. Now he has clear objectives: to lower blood pressure effectively and thereby to delay or prevent complication, in order to prolong life, and to provide maximum comfort and increased capacity to engage in the kind of work and activities that the patient prefers.

Moderate restriction of salt may be useful but it is no longer necessary to exist on a saltless, tasteless diet; it is no longer necessary to restrict the patient's work nor subject him to procedures that are dangerous or of dubious value. Contrast this with a statement made by an authority on hypertension in 1939:

Because an unproved *supposition* was held responsible for high blood pressure and kidney conditions, the patient was denied meat, especially red meat, which for some reason was regarded with particular dread. His diet was rendered even more disagreeable by the withdrawal of salt. Sympathy would doubtless have been extended to this half-starved fellow, except that he was probably unable to eat anyway, his teeth having been extracted on the theory that they *might* be infected and *infections might* have something to do with high blood pressure. Even before this, he had "sacrificed" his tonsils and had his sinuses punctured because of the same theory. In case some food had been consumed, enemas promptly washed out dangerous or poisonous substances from his bowels, a procedure which was enjoying a wave of popularity in those days.

If the patient was critically ill, bloodletting might be useful. This consisted of bleeding a patient from a vein, preferably in the bend of the elbow and allowing a pint or a pint and a half of blood to escape. It was hoped this would reduce high blood pressure. [I have personally measured the effect on high blood pressure by this procedure and found the pressure began to rise again in a few hours and was back at its pre-bleeding level the next day.]

To add to the patient's unhappiness, he was often told to stop work and exercise. Of course, he was denied alcohol and tobacco as well as coffee and tea, and, as a climax, he might have been separated from his sympathetic nervous system by a surgical operation which often produced only temporary reduction of the high blood pressure but left many painful and distressing side effects in its trail.

Although I have changed a word here and there and have inserted the result of some experiments I performed to find out what happened after bloodletting for high blood pressure, the sense of the message has not been altered. Such measures at one time were in general use. Mercifully, they have been virtually abandoned now. The methods we use today have been subjected to careful study and critical evaluation by independent and impartial scientists before they were recommended to the medical profession for general use. They are still being studied for improvement, and they undoubtedly will be further improved. A condensed version of two such studies is offered to show how medical procedures are now being checked and evaluated for the medical profession:

The first is from a recent, well conducted study by a team of expert physicians in Framingham, Massachusetts.

After they had studied thousands of people for several years, they concluded that elevated blood pressure had to be detected early and treated vigorously if strokes and other forms of brain damage were to be prevented. Blood pressure, by their standard, was considered too high if the systolic reached 160 or higher and the diastolic rose to 95 or higher. This applied to the two pressures, separately or together. A blood pressure above those levels is a risk, as I have mentioned before, because hypertension increases susceptibility to hardening of the arteries. I emphasize again that it is that risk factor rather than the height of blood pressure itself which it is necessary to prevent. Keeping the pressure within the normal range or as close to normal as possible is the best preventive.

That Framingham study also showed that physicians were mistaken when they thought that it is only or chiefly the diastolic pressure that held the dangerous risk factor; elevated systolic pressure carries as much a risk as the forerunner of a stroke or other complication, regardless of the patient's age. It had been widely held that mild hypertension in an older person was normal and harmless. I have told you that some rise in pressure is expected after 40 in each decade and that you were not to worry about it. That is so; do not worry about it, but do something about it: See your doctor. It is better to have the pressure brought under control. Besides he may find that the rise is associated with other symptoms which require attention.

Of particular interest was the conclusion of those investigators that in the elderly even mild hypertension in the absence of other symptoms may not be harmless. That is why taking the pressure has become routine in every physical examination during checkups, which one should have periodically at intervals of six months to a year. The recording of hypertension may indicate more frequent checkups for that purpose, because hypertension must be treated early and vigorously. Frequent visits enable the doctor to see whether the medication prescribed is working; if not, he will change it, because today he has a selection.

Another report issued from the Veterans' Administration likewise shows the preventive value of early and vigorous treatment. In a study of over 500 patients, observed from 20 months to over 3 years and longer, only 22 treated patients had complications; whereas among those who were not treated, complications developed in 56 cases, more than double. The investigators conducting that study were convinced that modern medical treatment of hypertension does effectively prevent complications. They recommended that treatment once started should be lifelong under periodic supervision by the physician, and that young patients with elevated pressure should submit to such supervision at once. Their experience bore out an observation made repeatedly, that elevated blood pressure was more serious among the black race than among the white.

The foregoing is intended to alert you, not to cause undue concern. Dangers have always been around us. If we recognize and understand some of them, we can take precautions. Hypertension is one danger which we can deal with effectively in modern times. Simple remedies are now available. Should one or two prove inadequate, we have a selection among a dozen others. A remedy ready for use will have the desired effect sought by you and your physician.

Treatment of High Blood Pressure: The New Pharmaceuticals

Doctors of old had not much to offer and they knew it. How happy they would have been if they had had such drugs as penicillin and a wide range of other antibiotics for infections; insulin, for diabetes, vitamin B_{12} for pernicious anemia; effective medicines to lower blood pressure. They did not even imagine the possibility of electric machines to start a heart beating again after it had stopped. Although they had medicines for use in high blood pressure, they knew that none was effective. In many ways, these are the good days, the "Good Old Days" were not medically good.

Thiazides are now the most useful medicines in the treatment of high blood pressure; they did not even exist until a comparatively few years ago. Their effects are twofold. First they increase the output of urine; hence the name *diuretic*. Second they lower blood pressure effectively; hence, they are called *antihypertensives*. The thiazides are especially effective in essential hypertension in which the primary aim is to lower blood pressure and thereby to delay or if possible to prevent complications. You will remember (page 23) that secondary hypertension is different, because the primary aim is to find the underlying cause of the *symptom* of hypertension. The thiazides can also be useful in treating and eradicating that form of hypertension by lowering the pressure and thus overcoming that one symptom of the underlying condition.

Thiazides have many advantages: They are effective when taken by mouth in the form of pills. The immediate lowering effect on blood pressure becomes apparent in less than an hour, and the effect of some preparations lasts from 3 to 6 hours. The patient must take the medicine three or four times a day to permit rapid adjustment in dosage at the outset of treatment if the condition is urgent. Other preparations are excreted more slowly; hence, their effects last longer and they need not be taken more than once or twice a day. Your doctor will select the preparation which is best for you. From time to time, he may change the preparation according to its current effectiveness.

Thiazides can also be used in conjunction with other blood pressure lowering medicines to induce what is called an *additive* effect, giving a greater and stronger response as each medicine adds to the total effect. Adverse side effects of thiazides are few and can be minimized easily or prevented by close supervision.

However, the output of urine, while draining off excessive fluid and sodium may, at the same time, deplete the amount of potassium essential to the body. Medications are available to block the loss of potassium, but it is also added as liquid. If your doctor prescribes a potassium pill, it will be one that is dissolved in water before taking. At the same time, your doctor will probably advise you to eat fruits high in potassium, such as bananas, cantaloupe, and orange juice. He may order periodic blood tests to study the percentages of the blood's chemical components, because the chemistry of the body must remain in balance as these medications are taken.

Treatment of Mild Hypertension

Chlorthiazide, one of the thiazide group of medicines, is frequently the medicine with which your doctor will start treatment. He may begin with some other member of the group, possibly with an ally of the thiazides. Be sure that he has a reason for choosing one preparation over another for you but allow him to make the choice.

It should be kept in mind that the thiazides and allied antihypertensive medicines are available under various trade names, according to the pharmaceutical company that makes them. They come in pill form and are usually given at the outset of treatment twice daily, after breakfast and after lunch, for a few weeks depending on the effect. When a satisfactory lowering of blood pressure has taken place, the dose can be reduced to one pill only, after breakfast, without loss of effect. This can reduce blood pressure significantly in more than two thirds of patients who have mild hypertension; but treatment must be maintained indefinitely under supervision of your doctor. Thiazides do not lose their effects on high blood pressure even when taken over long periods. On the other hand, the blood pressure tends to return to its previous elevated level when the medicine is discontinued.

Reserpine is an alternative medicine for the starting of treatment. It is less effective than a thiazide and more troublesome, because of its annoying side effects. The recommended initial dose is half a milligram daily for two to three weeks, subsequently reduced to a tenth or a fourth milligram daily. The doctor may have a reason for choosing this alternative to thiazide.

Full response to either reserpine or a thiazide is slow; it may require a few weeks. However, inadequate response to either medication does not mean that the dose should be increased. Larger amounts are not more effective and may induce unpleasant side effects. (This is especially true of reserpine.) Your doctor will probably start with a thiazide alone, but if reduction in blood pressure is inadequate, the next step is to add reserpine, which will give the good additive effect mentioned on page 52. The good effects of one are added to the good effects of the other, without inviting the unwanted side effects of larger doses of either. In the event of evidence of progressive rise of blood pressure or impending complication, more vigorous treatment may be necessary. Your doctor will know.

Moderately Severe Hypertension

The foregoing measures have been proved useful as a beginning for those who have never received treatment for high blood pressure. But if that preliminary treatment proves inadequate, thiazide and added reserpine are continued. Another medicine known as *hydralazine* is added, 10 milligrams twice a day at first, then slowly increasing to 25 to 50 milligrams three or four times a day. Your doctor will not permit you to use more than 200 milligrams a day; he will reduce the amount or stop it altogether after a few weeks, because he knows that it is inadvisable to continue large doses for a longer time.

Severe Hypertension

In severe hypertension, especially of long duration, treatment must be started cautiously, because hardening of the arteries affecting the heart, brain, or kidneys may already have begun. If reduction in blood pressure is too rapid or too abrupt, the patient's condition can be aggravated. That is why the effort is made to reduce the pressure gradually; restoration of blood pressure to normal levels is of secondary importance unless a reason to do otherwise is urgent. Reduction of blood pressure for those who do not yet have complications can prolong a useful life. Stronger medicines may be necessary and are available; however, in such instances, treatment is best carried out in a hospital, where the patient can be supervised more closely. The stronger medicines sometimes produce reactions requiring reduction in dosage or temporary discontinuance; the situation can be brought under control under hospital supervision.

What has been outlined is the method commonly followed by physicians. Your doctor may make some changes for a given patient because patients and circumstances differ. Your doctor can best decide that when examining you. What I have said so far, the procedure and the step-by-step examination, are intended to give you an idea of what to expect if you are a newcomer to such examinations. This is how it is done by physicians, with some likely modifications here and there. Emphatically, examination and treatment as described are not a do-it-yourself guide.

I have deliberately reversed the sequence by describing treatment before proceeding with the examination, the sooner to reassure you of the help awaiting you if you will seek it.

CHAPTER 8

How the Doctor Examines You and Why

Your Doctor Learns Basic Facts About You

The doctor learns the necessary facts about you by asking you many questions at the onset of your first interview. His questions are not prying, they are probing so that he may understand you and what is troubling you. A question about your age is significant in diagnosis, because some disturbances are likely at one age and some at another. Hypertension, for example, may come to teenagers, but it is almost always an occurrence of middle age and the later years. Tell the truth. Ladies, this is no time for coyness; besides, your doctor won't tell. Women often have hypertension during the change of life, although this may be a coincidence. Figures regarding hypertension expected at 50 would be alarming among adolescents.

The next question may be about your occupation, which has a great deal to do with the kind of life you lead. The doctor will ask about dusts, gases, or other harmful aspects of your work and living environments. If you have to bear heavy responsibilities, take risks, and make difficult decisions in the way an executive of a corporation must, then such tensions may have a bearing on your condition. At the opposite extreme, if you work as a lone wolf in building up a small business, that may also account for a number of factors. A harassed middle-aged mother with a cantankerous family may explain by that circumstance her condition. The doctor is not looking for gossip; he is not being impudently personal. He asks such questions because he is looking for clues to determine whether you are a likely candidate for the disorders of blood pressure. If your meals are hurried, your days anxious, and your nights broken by calls to duty, the doctor then understands that your difficulty may be heart trouble, blood pressure or stomach ulcers, common afflictions of those who lead hurried and harried lives. Some of the symptoms of hypertension are the same as those of heart trouble. Your doctor must find out which it is or whether it is neither. He does so by asking you more questions, observing you, and taking tests.

Your Family's Medical History: Heredity

Your parents' health and, if no longer living, what they died of, and sometimes even what your grandparents died of, will interest your doctor. Be patient and answer the questions as accurately as you can. He will also ask you about your brothers and sisters, particularly about their blood pressure. He is not wasting your time or his own with idle questions; they all have a point. Questions about your ancestors and other relatives may shed a great deal of light on your present discomforts. For one thing, we know that hypertension runs in families. If you inform him that your mother or father and one of their parents had high blood pressure, he will keep in mind that high blood pressure is a possibility in your case. On the other hand, your doctor will not make his diagnosis on that fact alone, and you are not to conclude that you have high blood pressure because someone in your family did. Although the condition runs in families, exceptions are many. Your doctor will use the information only as a clue.

Your Own Medical History

Your doctor will ask you to mention every illness you ever had from babyhood. He will ask also what other illnesses you are aware of having at the time of the interview. He will be particularly interested about rheumatic fever, diabetes, kidney trouble, and heart trouble.

Your habits are another probable topic, namely: Are you a cigarette smoker; if so, how many a day do you average? Or, how many cigars or pipefuls do you smoke in a day? Doctors have adopted an arbitrary maximum of 20 cigarettes daily. More than that is considered excessive and harmful. Whether fewer are safe is still an open question. Cigar smoking is considered less harmful and pipe smoking the least harmful. Perhaps it is because inhaling the smoke is greatest with cigarettes; it is less with cigars, and least with pipes. It is needless to explain to the doctor that you take only a few puffs on each cigarette and then discard it. If that is true (and in most cases it is not), experience shows that whether you take only a few puffs or smoke the entire cigarette, any number of cigarettes over 20 a day is certainly excessive and harmful.

Your doctor will also ask how many cups of tea or coffee you drink daily. He will want to know how much alcohol, especially hard liquor, you consume daily. If he thinks it appropriate, he might ask about use of such drugs as marihuana, heroin, or even LSD, especially if you are of the young generation.

Your Emotional Life

Your doctor will want to know about your daily routine; how you feel about your job and your associates, your married life, your children. He inquires about such things routinely, but the mention of headaches gives the matter a special importance. The doctor hears stories of far too many men and women to take an undue personal interest. His inquiries help him interpret what ails you. His attitude is professional toward everything you tell him and he holds it in sacred confidence, just as a priest does when hearing confession. Remember that a great many conditions, including hypertension, seem to go hand-in-hand with emotional stress and strain. Sometimes doctors think that those conditions may even be caused by anxiety and unhappiness, but whether this is so or not, we do not know. However, we do know that such conditions are made worse by worry. Personality and temperament always enter into the cause of illness. Even if a person's condition is due to causes that have nothing to do with one's own nature, such as being struck by lightning or a speeding truck, his emotions and outlook on life do influence the course and rapidity of recovery. When doctors see that the patient's answers often reveal only part of the truth, the patient makes it necessary for the doctor to rely on impressions more than on facts.

The Physical Examination

The direct history-taking having been concluded, your doctor then begins his thorough general examination, certainly including measurement of your blood pressure. If the pressure is higher than what is considered normal range at the given age (see page 14), he must determine whether the pressure is of the common variety, essential hypertension, for which there is no apparent cause; or, secondary hypertension, a symptom of some other underlying ailment which must be uncovered. Your doctor must make this distinction, for on it will depend the kind of treatment he will prescribe. I believe it necessary to repeat that essential hypertension requires treatment directed primarily to the high blood pressure itself, so as to delay or to prevent ultimate complications. If complications already exist, the doctor will treat the complications as well as the hypertension.

Secondary hypertension, as a symptom of something amiss with the kidneys or glands, or symptomatic of some other basic disease, must be dealt with as soon as possible. If the underlying cause of high blood pressure can be removed or controlled, the blood pressure may return to normal levels. If it does not thereby become lower, direct treatment of the blood pressure will be introduced.

Throughout his examination, the doctor studies your breathing. He observes whether it is normal or labored, regular or irregular, recurring in periodic cycles of increasing rate and depth of your respiration, then decreasing in depth and rate, perhaps followed by a moment or two of not breathing at all. Such periodic breathing has several possible causes, one being a faltering heart. If the doctor has reason to believe this possibility, he will at once look for additional clues, such as a bluish tint to the lobes of the ears or lips, the unduly distended veins at the sides of the neck which are hints that all is not well with your heart.

The doctor may ask if you have had dizzy spells or moments when you swayed or actually fell to the floor; or, if you have had temporary spells of weakness, loss of ability to move or use a limb, or loss of sensation in a limb. Such symptoms last from a few minutes to several hours, but as a rule, they clear up completely. Sometimes patients have temporary difficulty in speaking or in finding the right word they want to say. Your doctor inquires about such matters to find out if you had had warning symptoms of a stroke, the second important complication of high blood pressure; the more frequent is the impairment of the heart.

Less frequent are complications affecting the kidneys; therefore, you may be asked how many times you get up during the night to pass urine, whether you ever had kidney trouble, when your urine was last examined and what the results were, and whether chemical studies have ever been made of your blood to disclose whether your kidneys were functioning adequately.

The What, When, Why, and How of Your Pulse

The preliminaries over, your doctor will start with the actual physical examination. First, he will feel your pulse. The pulse can be felt in many places: in front of the ear, the side of the neck, in the groin, at the back of the knee joint, at the top of the foot, at the inner aspect of the ankle, and at other places where an artery runs just under the skin. As you probably know, the usual location where the pulse is taken is at the wrist, about 2 to 3 inches above the base of the thumb, at the outer margin of the lower end of the forearm. Does that sound a bit complicated? Not at all; you yourself will have no trouble in finding it once you are shown the actual location.

What the Pulse Is: The pulse is an abrupt, localized distention of the artery being felt, caused by the onward passage of blood through the arterial channel. It is felt by pressing a finger lightly over the artery when it runs close under the skin.

Why a Pulse: At the instant that the heart pumps its content of blood into the aorta, the beginning of the arterial system (see page 18, on the circulatory system), it distends that portion of the elastic artery. Backflow at that instant into the heart is prevented by closure of the heart valve. As the heart relaxes and backflow is prevented, the stretched aortic wall clamps down again, squeezing the blood forward. This, in turn, distends the next segment of the aorta or artery, which presently recoils elastically and pushes the blood farther onward. This process is repeated by each subsequent heart beat, giving rise to the *traveling pulse wave* which keeps pushing the blood toward its destination. This wave is what your doctor feels as the blood passes along the artery when he feels your pulse.

Rate: The doctor first counts the pulse rate per minute.

Since the pulse is originally generated by the heart beat, the rate of each is the same, unless the pulse wave is too weak by the time it reaches the wrist. The rate in the canary is about 1,000 beats a minute; in the elephant, it is about 25. The average normal rate in the adult human being is about 70 per minute, but as in the case of blood pressure, there is no absolute figure for normal. Anywhere between 60 and 90, a little more or less, per minute is in the average normal range.

A fixed normal rate is impossible to state because it varies among different persons. What is normal for one is not necessarily normal for another. The rate can normally be faster on walking, much faster after running, during excitement or nervousness, or after a meal. On the other hand, the rate may be slow and still be normal for that person. Napoleon was said to have had a pulse of 45, yet he was not a sick man until his final illness, which was cancer of the stomach.

Characteristics: In addition to counting the rate, the doctor observes whether the pulse wave has a rapid ascent and descent, whether it is "jerky," whether and what kind of irregularity is present, and the quality (or amplitude) of the wave, among other features.

It is interesting that ancient Egyptian documents mention philosophers and physicians of about 5,000 years ago who were aware of the pulse, counted it, and wondered about it. The difference today is that we count and observe it knowing what we are looking for; we understand the information that can be gained from that simple procedure.

Your Chest

Your heart and lungs are the most important organs in your chest; therefore, the doctor concentrates on them. He begins by tapping the chest and back by placing his open palm of the left hand snugly against your chest and striking the middle finger of his left hand with the end of the middle finger of his right hand, listening carefully to the sound thus produced.

What Tapping Tells About Your Lungs: If the sound is resonant and drumlike, your lungs are clear and full of air, as they should be if they are normal. A dense, dull, or flat sound suggests accumulation of fluid in your chest or some condition that prevents air from getting into your lungs, such as pneumonia or severe congestion, among other possibilities.

What Tapping Tells About Your Heart: The tapping begins at the extreme outer part of the left side of your chest. The doctor makes sure that he keeps tapping over the lung by listening for the tell-tale resonant sound. Your heart is a fleshy organ, containing blood, without air in any part of it. It is suspended in front of your left lung, and whenever the doctor taps over your heart, the sound is dull, not resonant as it is over the air-filled lung. He knows it is the heart and not the lung that is dull by its position. After beginning to tap toward the left, the doctor slowly moves his snugly applied left hand in a horizontal direction across the front of your chest, from left to right, without interrupting his tapping until he reaches the point where the sound changes abruptly from resonant to dull. That spot marks the location of the heart's left border.

The next step is to find out whether your heart is of normal size or is enlarged. If enlarged, the border will be too far to the left. Your doctor locates the mid-point of your left collar bone. From there, he drops an imaginary line straight downward. If the border of your heart lies to the right as he found it, or even at the downward line, the size of your heart is normal. If it extends toward the left beyond the line, your heart is enlarged. Observation through an instrument called the *fluoroscope* gives confirmation. If an even more accurate method still seems indicated, an x-ray of the chest settles any doubt.

Why does the doctor want to know the size of your

heart? Because your heart, which is a muscular pump, grows bigger when it has extra work to do like pumping blood into arteries where the pressure is high. That is all right for a time; but if the oversized job continues year after year, your heart enlarges and eventually has trouble keeping itself in order. Your doctor has all these in mind as he examines you.

What Does the Stethoscope Tell? Listening to your chest with a *stethoscope* is another important step toward diagnosis. The doctor places the end piece, a bell-shaped or flat disc, now here, now there, on your chest and back. It cuts out other noises, but brings the sounds produced in your lungs directly to the doctor's ears through its receiver and ear pieces. Crackling sounds mean congestion of the lungs; changes in quality of the breath sounds generally indicate bronchitis or inflammation in the lungs.

Tapping the chest and listening are simple tests; but to the experienced physician, they tell a great deal.

The doctor proceeds to listen with his stethoscope to your heart. Your heart is like a two-story duplex house with two rooms (chambers) upstairs and two downstairs (see Chapter 3, page 18). Blood flows in systematic fashion from one room to another within it and eventually out into your body and back again. The "doors" are the heart valves of the four chambers; while opening to admit the blood and then closing to prevent the backflow, they emit two soft sounds: lub-dub, lub-dub. Various cardiac (heart) disorders bring about changes in the rate, the rhythm and the quality of those sounds. These are what the doctor listens for with his stethoscope. Let us suppose for the time being that the doctor is satisfied with your heart and lungs. He must keep on looking for the cause of those headaches.

The Sphygmomanometer Measures Your Blood Pressure: The instrument that the doctor uses to measure your blood pressure has a jawbreaking name: sphygmomanometer. You have already seen the word here on page 36. It is pronounced: sfig'-mo-ma-nom'-i-tar, a word built up of three Greek words meaning pulse, thin, measure. The instrument measures blood pressure by means of a small column of fluid, customarily mercury. It looks like a room thermometer, but has a wide cloth cuff attached which your doctor wraps snugly around your arm above the elbow.

Blood pressure differs at different locations; it is highest at the aorta, the big artery you have read about here several times, the one by which the blood leaves the heart and begins the long circuit of the body. The brachial artery inside your arm is easy to reach and has become the conventional area for measurement. All doctors use it for this purpose; consequently, we can compare readings taken on different people, or on the same person taken at different times. Patients sometimes say: "I have hardening of the arteries; I am afraid the cuff of the apparatus will have to be squeezed too hard to register my blood pressure and will reach a figure higher than it really is." However, arteries are elastic tubes. Even if they have become hardened, they will yield to the cuff's squeezing. This point has been checked scientifically in several ways. We know that hardening of the arteries does not interfere with measurement of blood pressure as it is now practiced.

How Blood Pressure Was First Measured: Blood pressure was first measured in 1733 by Stephen Hales, an English clergyman with a scientific turn of mind. He inserted a long glass tube in an artery of a horse and measured the height to which the column of blood rose within the tube. This was hardly a suitable method for human use. Many devices for measuring human blood pressure were then suggested, but none was satisfactory until Riva-Rocci, an Italian scientist, constructed a model type of instrument in 1896. That instrument was practical, free from objectionable features, and accurate enough to meet all requirements. It is now in use by physicians all over the world, the sphygmomanometer. Riva-Rocci recognized that if you find out how much it takes to stop the flow of blood in your artery, you then know what the blood pressure is, for the two are the same. His instrument stopped the flow by compression of the arm—it was substantially the same as the instrument used today: a rubber bag wrapped like a cuff around the patient's arm and then inflated until it presses hard enough to stop the circulation.

In 1905 a Russian physician, Korotkow, practicing in what was then called St. Petersburg, introduced a refinement. He used a stethoscope with the apparatus. He laid the "bell" or flat disc of the endpiece of the stethoscope over the patient's artery at the bend of the elbow, just below the cuff, and listened for changes in the sounds as the blood supply was cut off. He was thus able to note the height of the blood pressure of both the working heart (systolic pressure) and of the resting heart (diastolic pressure).

Measuring Your Systolic Blood Pressure (Figure 1, facing page): Now you will understand what the doctor

FIGURE 1. (on facing page) *A sphygmomanometer.* The cuff (C) which contains a flat rubber bag is applied snugly around the arm. The valve (V) is closed so that air can be pumped into the bag but none can escape. Air is then forced into the bag by alternately compressing and releasing the bulb (B). The bag becomes distended as the air pressure within it is increased, thus constricting the arm to any desired degree. The increased air pressure within the bag is also transmitted through the other tube into a small reservoir (MR) which contains mercury. The mercury is thus forced up into the glass tube (GT) and the height in millimeters to which the mercury rises is measured on the scale (S). The method of measuring the systolic and diastolic blood pressures is described in the text.

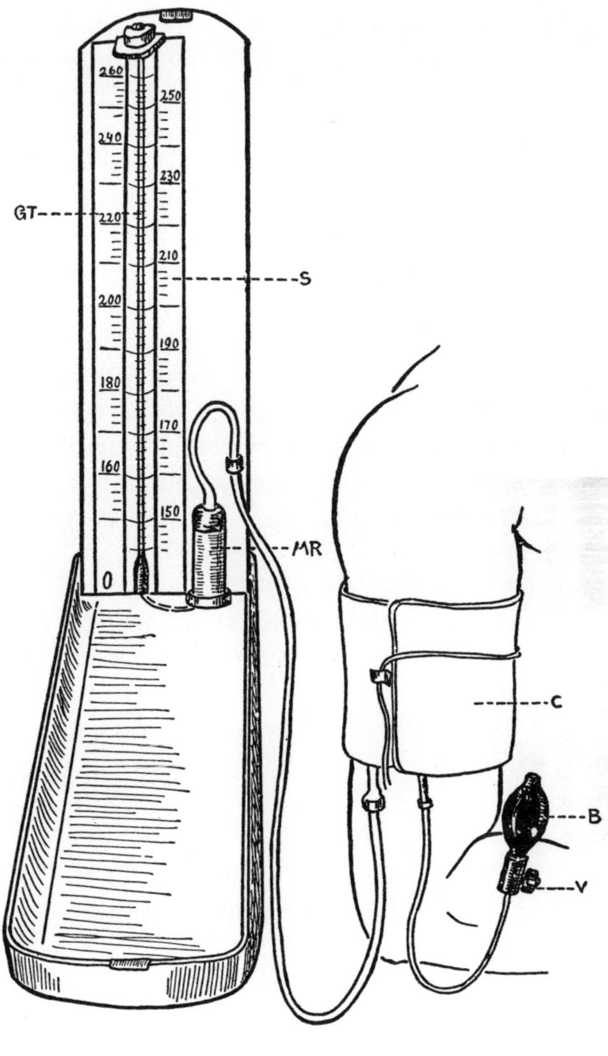
GT
S
MR
C
B
V
260
250
240
230
220
210
200
190
180
170
160
150
0

is doing when he winds the cloth cuff around your arm to measure your blood pressure. The cloth cuff is just a case containing a rubber bag. The doctor pumps it up like a bicycle tire by squeezing a rubber ball attached to it by tubing. A second tube joins the rubber bag to the upright board, to which the manometer (the glass tube containing mercury) is screwed. The doctor pumps up the bag until it squeezes hard enough on your flesh to stop the blood briefly in your brachial artery. He knows when that point has been reached by listening at the bend of your elbow with his stethoscope as Korotkow did. He pumps until the sounds of your pulse can no longer be heard. Then, listening all the while, he slowly lets the air out of the bag. You should not talk to him during this procedure, for the sounds he wants to hear are not loud; he must give them his closest attention. He releases the pressure on your arm gradually until he can hear the first sounds of the returning pulse as the blood rushes back into the compressed area of your arm.

The doctor makes a note at this moment of the height of the mercury in the tube as shown on the scale marks alongside the tube. The pressure in your artery is the amount of pressure it took to push the mercury to the height in the tube while your heart was in its *working phase*. The figure the doctor makes a note of is your systolic blood pressure.

Measuring Your Diastolic Blood Pressure (Figure 2): To learn the pressure in your brachial artery *while your heart is relaxing between its contractions*, or beats, your doctor blows up the bag a second time, while he continues to listen through the stethoscope. Again he deflates the bag until a change in the sounds tells him that the blood is beginning to return to that part of your arm. At this time, he keeps on letting the air out of the bag slower, and the mercury in the glass tube keeps on dropping slower. Even-

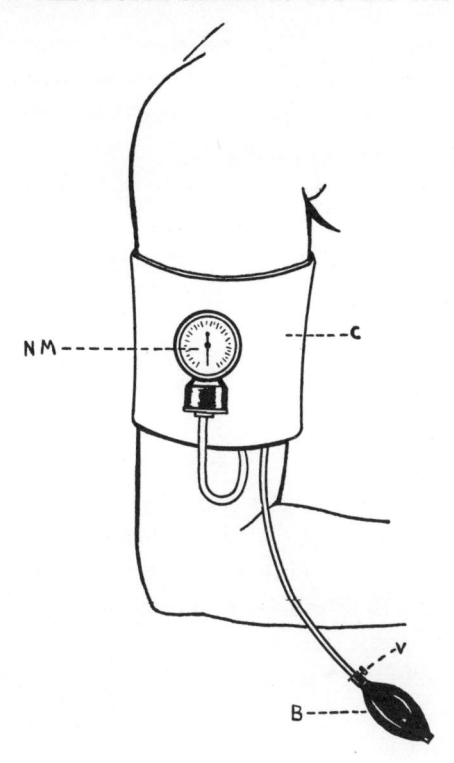

FIGURE 2. *Another type of sphygmomanometer.* Here the pressure is indicated by a needle which revolves like the hand on the face of a clock. NM is needle manometer.

tually the clear tones brought by the stethoscope to the doctor's ears stop altogether. That is when he notes the height of the mercury: that figure is your *diastolic pressure.* Suppose the reading is 90; it means that to overcome the resistance to the flow of blood offered by your arteries, your heart must give a push great enough to lift the mercury 90 millimeters, or a little under 4 inches, up the tube.

Your diastolic pressure is always a lower figure than your systolic, for it is the measure of force in the split second between one beat and the next when your heart is taking a respite from work. If either number is above the average range for your age and sex, your doctor will know that you are hypertensive and will go from there to find out why. Your blood pressure has given him the first objective clue toward solving the reason for your symptoms. If he now knows that you have hypertension, it confirms his original impression based on your frequent early morning headaches, so characteristic of high blood pressure.

The Urine Tests

If you have ever given any thought to the matter, you must realize that urine, like many body discharges, is medically interesting because it provides some evidence of conditions inside your body; it carries messages from within. Each message is interpreted by means of an appropriate test. That is why the doctor asks for a sample of urine, which the laboratory technician analyzes. It is probable that the doctor will ask you to bring along a small specimen of urine in a bottle, the first urine passed after you get up in the morning. The reason for that is that during the night you normally do not drink, so that solids and other elements in the urine are less diluted than they are later in the day when urine becomes fairly diluted by the fluids taken.

Albumin: In the laboratory, part of the specimen is drawn off and put through a chemical test for *albumin*, a substance that sometimes, but not always, carries the message that something is amiss. Albumin is a protein produced during digestion of your food and is used by the body to restore old cells and build new ones. (The cells are the basic units, or "building blocks," of your body.) Albumin is too valuable a material for your body to lose, and therefore it does not appear in the urine under normal conditions. However, if your kidneys are impaired by some infection or in some other way, albumin will appear in all likelihood in the urine; that is, traces of the albumin will be eliminated in the urine. Your doctor will proceed to discover why. The kidneys are discussed at length in the chapter on secondary hypertension, Chapter 11, page 107.

Let me emphasize before leaving the topic of albumin that its presence is not an absolute sign of something wrong, but your doctor will want to make sure, reserving his conclusion until further tests show whether the kidneys are indeed infected or damaged.

Nephritis: Nephritis is also known as Bright's disease, after the nineteenth-century London physician Richard Bright. At first nephritis was thought inevitably fatal. Bright himself was able to accumulate evidence that the ailment was not so dangerous as at first believed. Antibiotics have largely overcome its early fear-instilling outlook. (See further discussion of nephritis, page 109.)

Casts: The doctor next looks for signs of kidney damage: the presence of *casts* or blood in the urine. Casts are clumps of dead cells, the product of infection or another disturbance, which plug up the tiny tubes in the kidneys. Casts are so called because they take their rodlike shape from the tubes, like a plaster cast. But the casts are also not *always* a signal of something wrong. The test is conducted as follows: the sediment in the urine is obtained by a centrifuge process, and is then examined under a microscope to determine whether casts and blood cells are present. The patient may pass this test as well.

Kidney's Efficiency: The doctor then tests for the kidneys' efficiency. The kidneys have two responsibilities: to collect fluids and soluble wastes of the body (the bowels attend to the solid matter) and to dilute them for convenient elimination by way of the bladder. If the kidneys cannot fulfill their responsibilities, the urine they produce will not be so fully loaded with waste products as it should be, so that such products remain in the body instead of being discarded. If that is the case, *renal function tests* (tests of the kidneys' function and the region around them) become necessary. A tiny instrument is floated in the urine; if it rides high on the surface, the urine is highly concentrated; if it sinks low, the urine is carrying a light load. If you take this test and pass it, it remains to be seen whether the kidneys are providing liquids for flushing off the waste they collect. To do this, the patient must drink about a quart and a half of fluid. During the next four or five hours, if the kidneys are working well, the patient should void nearly all of it in the form of thin diluted urine.

Other ingenious tests for renal function are available. The important point is that when kidneys are impaired, the waste that they fail to remove accumulates in the blood. This causes discomfort, but that discomfort is a warning signal of something within requiring attention. Heed that warning immediately. By examining the urine and, at the same time, samples of the blood, the doctor can come to a fair conclusion about what is happening. He will then determine by chemical tests whether there is an excess of urea, creatinine, nonprotein nitrogen, and other substances in the blood which give evidence that the kidneys are not being efficient.

Kidneys may also be examined by x-ray; the resulting picture is called a *pyelogram,* about which you may read more on page 111.

Examining Your Eyes

All the kidney tests may have justified the doctor's discarding any theory he may have had about renal or kidney disorder. He has one way left to explain your headaches and essential hypertension. We know from autopsies (examinations of the body after death) what hardened arteries look like. We have one open window through which to see arteries in life: the eyes, and that is why they are examined (Figure 3). When examining your eyes because of hypertension, your doctor is not testing for glasses. He is simply looking for the only sample of your arteries accessible to him. He reasons that what he sees there is a fair idea of what he would see in your other arteries were

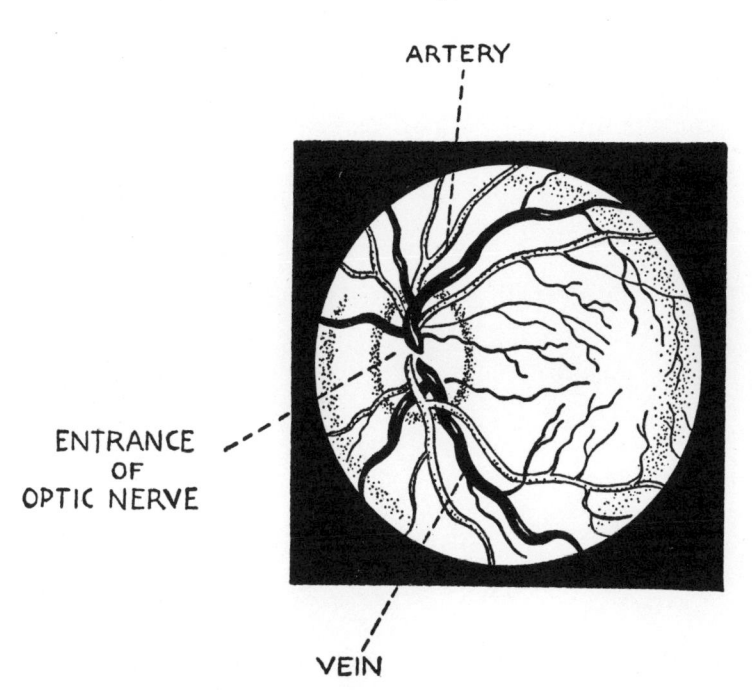

FIGURE 3. *What your doctor sees when he examines the inside of the eye with an ophthalmoscope.* The circular area near the center is the optic nerve as it enters the eye. This is the nerve of vision. Small veins and arteries issue from this area like spokes of a wheel. Your doctor can see the condition of these vessels and from them he often gets a clue about the probable condition of the arteries in other regions.

he able to see them. The doctor may be satisfied that the diagnosis of essential hypertension fits all the facts and observations made in your case. Your eyes may have told him that a degree of hardening of the arteries is present as a consequence of the pressure that the arteries have been called on to withstand as your blood pushes through your body (Figures 4 and 5).

CHAPTER 9

WHAT YOU CAN DO FOR YOURSELF

Let me say again that until we know the cause of essential hypertension, we can treat only symptoms—but you should not therefore underestimate the importance of treating the symptoms and bringing the pressure down and under control to prevent or delay complications; the sooner this is done, the better the chance for successful treatment. We keep finding better and better ways, and we now have better medicines for lowering high blood pressure. The ideal is to prevent hypertension from taking place; but this calls for understanding of the fundamental cause of the disorder, and this we still await from medical researchers who are at work on the problem. We have learned how to make people less susceptible to the development of high blood pressure. Physicians now add comfortable years of life to the nation's hypertensive population. If you follow your doctor's directions carefully, so far as essential hypertension goes, you can enjoy a long and useful existence. It is not at all rare now for men and women with essential hypertension to live out their normal years, long after the condition was first recognized. Those are the men and women who did not neglect treatment after recognition of the disorder and who did for themselves what is possible for hypertensive patients to do.

Statistics become largely meaningless at this point, because no one knows how long a hypertensive person had high blood pressure before it came to light. No one can say for sure what the outlook is, because we usually do not know when it began. However, we do know that it is not how high the pressure is that determines in itself the outlook; the condition of the arteries determines the outlook. We have been keeping records about hypertensive people for so many years. Since we have had the sphygmomanometer, measuring blood pressure during every physical examination has become routine practice. We have learned that three out of four patients with essential hypertension, when their time comes, die *not* because of the high blood pressure but of entirely different, unrelated disorders. No one would choose to have hypertension, but it is certainly among the least that can befall one, provided that it is not neglected. Has earlier recognition and modern treatment greatly improved the outlook?

Studies have shown that even modest elevations of either systolic or diastolic pressure, in the long run, do increase mortality rates. However, modern antihypertensive treatment, even of mild hypertension, is associated with longer and improved survival; hence, the importance of early and modern treatment *has been proved*. In the light of what we now know, elevations in blood pressure—even when moderate, of the systolic blood pressure and without symptoms—should be treated with our modern medicines in order to bring down the pressure to normal limits and avoid its risks. This is what good preventive medicine means. You may continue with your work, as long as it is not too strenuous for your age, and your play. If you have symptoms, your doctor will give you advice on how to live, supplemented by procedures which he will perform for you. But this much, you can do for yourself:

Rest and Relaxation to Help Yourself

Your blood pressure may be brought within normal limits by rest and relaxation. It is worth a trial, as a start, in mild cases in which the pressure fluctuates and the rise does not last long. When you sleep or lie down for a rest period, you ease your heart and arteries and your blood pressure falls. The condition is more serious if the blood pressure rises too high and stays there. Going to bed for about ten days sometimes puts an end to headaches, fatigue, dizziness, tenseness, and the shortness of breath. The blood pressure thus goes down bit by bit. Or, your doctor may find it wise to add the newer blood pressure lowering medicines to speed the process. After about ten days, the pressure should remain at a level significantly lower than when you took to bed. You can then continue with your medicine, get up, and resume your normal life.

It is more difficult but highly important to follow the obligation to relax. This you must do, above all else. Hypertensive persons are often worriers, although they try to mask the trait. Some think life has cheated them, and resent that others seem to live on a bed of roses; however, they forget about the thorns. Sometimes troubles are real, but often they are of one's own making. Reasons for tension are all about us, yet we must train ourselves to cope with them.

You may think it is easy for the doctor to sit on the other side of the desk from you and tell you to stop worrying. But you are not the first patient he has ever advised. He knows his orders are hard to follow. He has had to learn to do this himself. He knows even more surely that you had better follow them if you want to live.

Many business and professional men, especially if they have worked up from the very bottom, will not relax. They are afraid to let go of the tiger's tail. They are difficult patients and hard to manage, because they accomplish so much in other matters but can't overcome hypertension in their own way. Women who are perfectionists about their many cares may be equally difficult to hold in line.

On the whole, women are more cooperative with their physicians than men; they follow advice as well as they can.

About Spas

European doctors are greater believers in mineral water spas than are American doctors. In this country such resorts as Saratoga Springs, White Sulphur Springs, Hot Springs, French Lick, Colorado Springs, and others seem to have continually full houses. When my patients ask me if a health resort would help them, I tell them that if they can lead a regular sensible life and put their worries behind them or aside, it does not matter whether they go away or stay at home. What makes people feel better at health resorts is only in part the drinking of the mineral water or the local warm baths. Of far more benefit are the pleasant surroundings, the stimulation of a new place and new friends, and the simple fact of being out of reach, more or less, of the telephone, the ticker tape, the loudspeaker, the foreman, the boss, the time clock, and for some, even the friends and relatives. If you take driving, nagging, guilt-provoking presences with you in your mind, then stay at home, save your money and spend it on learning to relax, if you can. The Africans in their jungle huts and the South Sea Islanders on their paradise-beaches do not know about high blood pressure. If you go there and seek the same sun and do get better, it will not be because of the paradise, but because you sloughed off your worries when you packed your luggage. If you go but do not get better, it will be because you did not slough off your cares.

For most men and women, who cannot afford to leave everything behind and devote themselves full-time to a cure, certain compensations are possible: "Better a dinner of herbs where love is than a stalled ox and hatred therewith," was Solomon's way of pointing out the vanity of material possessions and the blessing of love and happiness. If we doctors could prescribe domestic peace and a contented mind as easily as we prescribe pills, we could cure an impressive percentage of patients tomorrow. Meanwhile, a sensible substitute for a long trip is to take a little vacation *every day*, or some other little "pause that refreshes" when you can best arrange it.

Is Sexual Abstinence Necessary?

Sexual intercourse is not prohibited for patients with controlled essential hypertension; but you must make sure that you do not have any complications of hypertension and that such complications are not impending. How can you make sure? Discuss it with your doctor. Blood pressure is increased during intercourse, but the rise is of short duration and generally does not induce harmful effects *in the absence of complicating conditions*. Undue shortness of breath, tightness or pain in the chest or excessive fatigue after the exertion are signs that the strain has been too great. It is the same as having similar symptoms at other times, such as on climbing a flight of stairs or walking a few blocks, or during any type of excitement.

Abstinence is recommended if any of the symptoms mentioned develop. Your doctor will recommend abstinence if your heart is faltering, or you have warning signals that your brain is not receiving a normal supply of blood, or that your kidney function is impaired. Do not make the decision yourself. Ask your doctor and abide by his advice; otherwise, you may be practicing unnecessary restraint or disregarding signals and so invite trouble. Your doctor may advise you to abstain until your blood pressure has been reduced and the symptoms have been brought under control.

What About Pregnancy?

During pregnancy, it is not at all uncommon for even young women to become hypertensive, although that may be the only occurrence in their lives. Usually, it is some other cause, such as a kidney disorder, which gives trouble. If pregnancy is not watched and any untoward condition corrected, it can be a hazard. If the urine is normal and the level of essential hypertension is not high, the outlook for the woman and the baby is good. Each pregnancy must be regarded as a separate event, however, and the woman must not judge it by the preceding one. The duration of each pregnancy must be closely watched by the doctor from beginning to end, and with your cooperation, the doctor can maintain the pressure at a safe level by diet and medication.

Fighting Fatness

The medical profession is beginning to regard obesity as something close to a harmful disease. That may not be strictly accurate; but there is no doubt whatever that it makes you an easy prey to any one of a wide variety of illnesses—including hypertension. If you are ill, being fat delays your recovery and lessens your prospects of survival.

You will understand what fatness does to your frame and your organs if you think of it as a heavy burden from which you are never free. You may sink into a chair to take the weight off your feet, but what about your heart? Your heart never takes a holiday, never has a rest period (except between beats). However, if you are overweight, you force it to pump more blood farther in order to nourish your overstuffed chassis. And what of your bones and muscles that must support your excessive flesh? What of your legs and feet, which have to hold you up and carry you around? Fatty tissue grows in your heart muscle also, hampering it in its vital work. Not only that, as fat accumulates, your oversized abdomen encroaches on the space in your chest and pushes up your heart. When you overeat, you actually push your heart around. You pay the price of fatness in ways you cannot see. Isn't that reckless and unintelligent?

What of your personality? It may not be true that nobody loves a fat man, but certainly nobody envies him. Whoever said to a fatty, "How did you do it?" Everyone knows. He eats too much. But if you can discipline yourself for the next few months, or better still, for the next year or two, you will have the joy of hearing your friends ask you, "How did you do it? I wish I could." You can. Anyone can. And if you are a hypertensive person, a heart patient, a diabetic or almost anything else, *you had better*. Not only will you be healthier, but you will also be happier. Discipline yourself to lose weight.

Insurance statistics prove that obesity costs life. That is why applications for insurance always ask your weight. For men and women who weigh 10 pounds over the ideal weight for their age, the death rate is 8% above the normal death rate. For those who are 20 pounds too heavy, the death rate rises to 18%. Those whose weight is 30 pounds too much have a death rate 28% above the average, and it mounts to 56% if the excess is 50 pounds. These are depressing facts. Let me translate them into the story of Mrs. X, one of my saddest patients.

Mrs. X was (not is) a middle-aged housewife under 5 feet in height who weighed over 200 pounds. Her face and lips were bluish as she waddled with difficulty into my office. Her complaints were many, including persistent cough and difficulty in getting her breath. She tired easily. When she was told that her blood pressure was high, she came to see me.

I found her lungs congested; an electrocardiogram showed the effects of heart strain. Her systolic blood pressure fluctuated at around 200 and her diastolic, at around 120. Her legs were swollen and puffy; the veins in her neck bulged from congestion. She looked as if she were angry; as a matter of fact, she had a violent temper which she always vented on those about her in the belief that she had plenty of provocation. Her business did not run smoothly and was a source of anxiety. Her relatives gossiped too much and her children would not do as she wished. Most exasperating of all was her daughter-in-law who was actually proposing to move out and run her own home.

Mrs. X indulged in two outlets for her nervousness. She smoked up to 80 cigarettes a day and ate almost unceasingly. She told me that she consumed three good-sized meals a day and an extra dinner at midnight, not to mention the snacks she had to have when she was angry—which was most of the time. More than once she got herself into such a state that she had to give up and go to a hospital. There it was not so hard for her to diet. She was watched closely; no one was allowed to smuggle in food. She had no choice. She could lose between 3 and 5 pounds a week, sometimes more, and even that small amount would lower her blood pressure somewhat. If we could have kept this up, she would probably be alive now and happier. But she was her own worst enemy. After a couple of weeks in the hospital, she always found it necessary to get out. She became restless; she knew her affairs were going awry without her and her daughter-in-law was up to no good—bringing up the grandchildren all wrong and probably giving her beloved son the wrong things to eat.

I did my best to tell her how dangerous her course of living was, and she, in turn, promised that she would now eat less, stop smoking, and control her temper. Of course, she never did, and her shortness of breath increased as her huge bulk pressed on her abused heart at the same time that the bulk demanded more work from the heart. Her incessant smoking caused incessant coughing, and that added to the strain on her heart and the labor of breathing. Her heart began to show unmistakable signs of faltering. Her family phoned one evening in a state of alarm, because the patient had a violent headache and was in extreme distress. The patient died of a massive stroke on the way to the hospital.

Mrs. X had made all the possible mistakes. Although many contributing habits and their results entered into her story, weight alone would have brought about the same inevitable result. A doctor knows that he is licked before he starts when an overweight patient is uncooperative, since he cannot rid the patient of the excess weight. This the patient must do for himself. By way of contrast, let me tell you how another patient did it.

A 19-year-old young lady, a college freshman, consulted me for obesity. She was about 4 feet, 10 inches tall, and weighed 147 pounds. She had been under the care of another physician who had prescribed 10 grains of thyroid daily, an unusually large amount. Her weight did not change appreciably and she was unable to adhere to a weight-reducing diet. Physical examination showed nothing abnormal. There was no evidence of thyroid inadequacy or other glandular disorder. It was obvious that the girl was having psychological difficulties, and was eating too much as a compensation. During an interview, she told of her difficulty with her school work, although her grades were excellent. She was unpopular—had no social life, and no dates with young men. She was certain that her parents would consider her a failure.

I explained to the patient that being overweight in her case was not due to some physical deficiency; she did not have thyroid or other glandular disturbance, and did not need thyroid medication. I emphasized the truth and value of the traits that she did have, namely an attractive personality, excellent character, better than average deportment, and better than average performance in her school studies. I argued that her real troubles stemmed from an unwarranted feeling of insecurity, self-deprecation, and uncalled-for defeatism. I suggested that perhaps a change in environment would be helpful, as well as some reassurance and help from a sympathetic person on whom she could rely and who would bring her a taste of social success. I suggested that her brother might be such a person. He attended a large college elsewhere and, being on good terms with him, she transferred there. Because she was an art major, I suggested that she might exploit that talent. The patient's brother did open the gates for her to a more active social life. Thus motivated, she overcame her compulsion to eat too much; her weight dropped from 147 and remained at 97 pounds. Her painting improved to the point where she received many invitations to exhibit her work. She became a well-known artist, and a well-adjusted mate and housewife.

That patient had a happy outcome. It is interesting to reflect what might have happened had her weight not been brought under control. Her mother had hypertension and died of one of its complications. Her sister and other relatives had hypertension. With that family history, she was certainly a candidate for high blood pressure. Obesity only added another high risk. It is highly probable that the altered life pattern overcame those predisposing factors. After twenty years and four children, she still has a normal blood pressure.

The Mathematics of Losing Weight: Life insurance company statistics indicate that about 20,000,000 people in the United States are 10% or more overweight. We can see from these statistics that obesity is a health problem. Overweight alone contributes to the development of heart ailments, high blood pressure, advanced hardening of the arteries, gallbladder disease, diabetes, and arthritis in weight-bearing joints. It increases the risk in surgical operations and favors formation of blood clots in veins and arteries.

Being overweight places a heavy burden on the heart. A pound of fat tissue contains about two-thirds of a mile of blood vessels and the heart has to pump that much more blood in order to nourish that 1 pound of useless fat. When you eat more than your body requires, the excess food is converted into useless fat and is stored in that form.

Familial environment is important in becoming overweight. A study has shown that about 82% of obese women had one or both parents who were overweight. Another study showed that if both parents were fat, 73% of their children also became overweight. If only one parent was fat, 59% of the children were overweight. Only 9% of their children were overweight when both parents had normal weight. For the sake of your children and your own health do not overeat to the point of becoming obese. If your daily program of activity takes less energy than your food intake supplies, you will put on weight. If your daily program uses up more energy than your food intake yields, you will lose weight. Eat just enough to supply your energy requirements in order to maintain a normal weight.

At the back of this book, you will find a table of normal weights for your sex and height which will set your goal. A program of reducing diets is also provided, one yielding about 1,000 calories and another about 1,500 calories. You will not need to count calories; these are examples of balanced diets easily obtained anywhere, and they are pleasant. All you need to do is to heed the specified amounts; you must watch quantity, not calories as such. If you have allergies to any of the foods suggested, or if some other condition that you have makes substitutions desirable, talk them over with your doctor. These diets consider calories *only*, in order to reduce weight. They may have to be modified for other reasons.

Reducing weight is simply a problem of mathematics. In the course of the day you burn up food to get energy, just as a furnace burns fuel to give off heat. If you lie in bed, the acts of breathing, digesting, eliminating, looking, thinking, talking, all require energy, and the energy derived from a certain fraction of what you eat will supply the need. Normally, you do more than that. You move about, walk, climb stairs, cook dinner, dress the baby, dictate letters, fill out forms, drive the car, play tennis, swim, pack your luggage, carry your golf bags, and so on. With every effort that you make in the day, and every turnover in bed you make at night, you draw on energy over and above the minimal basic requirements. Your energy comes from your digested food. Although every act of living takes up some energy, most people eat more than they need for the energy expended.

A diet of 1,000 to 1,500 calories a day usually results in loss of 1 or 2 pounds a week, if you are moderately active. Unless you are grossly fat, that is a sufficiently rapid reduction. Do not deceive yourself that snacks do not count. They may be the core of your problem. A small chocolate bar furnishes you from 200 to 250 calories. A chocolate malted milk or one serving of pie gives you 450 calories. That alone is more than one-fourth to one-half of all the calories you should have in the day if you wish to reduce. A good general rule is to cut down drastically on the starches, the sugars, and the fats. Study a chart of calories to see where these ingredients are hidden. Soft drinks, for example, are fattening to the degree of their sugar content. Alcoholic beverages are fattening, because alcohol is fattening. If you must drink those beverages, then be sure to whittle down somewhere else, so that you do not go beyond the day's total allowance of calories. If you must have a snack at bedtime, save something from dinner. More important than what you eat or how much you eat of one food or drink is your staying within your daily caloric limits; however, it is wise to make your selection so as to have a balanced diet *within your allowance of calories.*

Appetite Suppressants: Your doctor will probably hesitate to prescribe a medication to depress your appetite, because the medicine becomes a psychological crutch on which you may all too easily learn to lean. The goal calls for self-discipline. Govern yourself, control your appetite, and the surplus weight will go.

For the sake of complete coverage, I will mention that medicine is available to reduce weight but it is of temporary benefit and does not permanently eradicate the cause. In short, such medicines are not a cure. They are used chiefly, if at all, at the beginning of treatment to suppress appetite and to help the patient at his most difficult time to adhere to a reduced food intake.

Thyroid was popular for many years as a weight-reducing agent. But most obese persons have normal thyroid function. The amount necessary to reduce weight varies with different people. Moderate amounts are seldom adequate; and fairly often, results are not obtained until toxic doses are used. However, such amounts can be dangerous and, at best, do not get at the cause of overweight, which is *overeating.* (Forgive my saying this so often. It is the best word you can take away from reading this book if losing weight is a necessity for you.)

Chief medical reliance today is on the amphetamines, of which dexedrine is an example. It is taken in small amounts about half an hour before meals to suppress appetite. Adjustments may be necessary from time to time; hence, the drug should be used if at all *only under the supervision of your physician.* It may interfere with sleep, in which case, omission of the evening dose, before dinner, may be necessary. The regular amount is taken for about 2 weeks of dietary treatment, after which the dosage is reduced gradually over the next 3 weeks. By that time, the patient should be accustomed to the smaller food intake of a reducing diet.

I would like to think that persons with high blood pressure who have enough insight to read how they can help themselves will cooperate with their physicians in exercising self-control in their eating habits, and will be strong enough in their determination to manage without the dubious crutch of appetite-depressing medication. I would especially like to think that my readers here would not be gullible to the lures of patent medicines that purport to reduce weight. There are two aspects to weight reduction; you must lose weight, and re-educate your eating habits, so that you will not regain the weight that you have lost. The rewards come at once. Your blood pressure falls, keeping pace with your reducing. Your friends' admiration and even envy will be sweet; you will look better, feel better, and your clothes will even fit better. Movements that you could hardly manage before become easy: bending, running, kneeling. And you may want to kneel, in thankfulness.

Food Fads: Freak diets that concentrate on one food to be eaten or not to be eaten are not ideal, and may even be harmful. Almost every common food has at one time or another been considered the cause of high blood pressure. It was fashionable some years ago to attribute high blood pressure to meat. Yet, Stefansson, the polar explorer, lived nine years on seal meat and water and never had high blood pressure. We know more now about how food is utilized in the body and we are convinced that meat should not be neglected as it contains protein, a builder of needed tissue, and is an enormous appetite quencher.

Ever since 1904, when a French physician pronounced

that blood pressure could be brought down by eliminating salt from food, the salt-free diet has been periodically in vogue. We seem to be in the midst of another revival of the doctrine that salt deprivation will put an end to hypertension; however, neither science nor experience supports this view, although there may be collateral reasons for prescribing a low sodium diet. Salt substitutes, in cases in which low sodium is indicated, can relieve the tastelessness, and improvements have generally removed the metallic taste of these substitutes. Only about one of every 10 hypertensive persons can tolerate the tediousness and tastelessness of unsalted food for any length of time. And yet it must be strictly maintained for a lifetime to prevent a recurrence of high blood pressure. Many people feel weak and listless without salt; it appears that we are like cattle, who will go miles to a salt lick, and need it in some vital fundamental way. With modern medication, the diuretic draws off the salt, so that the diet need not be pallid.

The fat-free diet is a trying diet. Fat does add calories and consequently, weight; however, the reasoning on which the fat-free diet is based is not clear. We know that hardening of the arteries is common, more so in men and women who have hypertension than among those whose pressure is normal. But we do not know how or why hypertension makes one more susceptible to hardening of the arteries. We continue to stress that gap in our understanding. Reliable evidence that fat causes hypertension is at hand, only indirectly: namely that too much fat may make you overweight. That is the inducing factor in hypertension.

Your Beloved Bad Habits: Many patients ask me about their favorite indulgences, commonest of which are tobacco, coffee, tea, and alcohol. My advice is just stop smoking; do not try to taper off. Those patients often reply that if they did not smoke they would eat more. They may, if they do not learn to control themselves. Filtered and denicotinized cigarettes are still tobacco, whatever the advertisers say, even if the cigarettes do contain less nicotine and other undesirable substances. There is too much evidence accumulating to ignore the caution that tobacco in any form is harmful in one way or another. Alcohol in any form is best avoided. Remember that alcohol is also very fattening. Tea and coffee taken with cream or sugar or both add calories; they are stimulants, but one or two cups of either a day will not harm you. Do not use those stimulants to spur yourself to make efforts when you are already fatigued. You will be really punishing yourself if you do. If a coffee break helps you to relax, you can get the same effect from one of the caffein-free products.

Spot Weight Reduction: There is no scientific evidence that spot weight reduction, whether of the hips, the buttocks, the legs, or any other location, can accomplish anything worthwhile.

Milk Farms

Milk farms are in the same category as freak diets, such as those demanding that the patient eat only rice or only "Nature" foods. The American Medical Association has reported on the extreme danger to health that lies in the so-called Zen diet, a "far out" example of the Nature cult.

The milk farms (as any drastic intake of one food to the exclusion of all others, and then only on a highly restricted basis) most certainly will reduce weight, but they are temporary and spectacular expedients. They can be unpleasant, troublesome and often harmful. Shortly after the so-called treatment is over, the patient resumes his former eating habits and the lost weight is regained quickly. What is the sense in losing 40 pounds during several weeks or months of unpleasantness only to regain it all in half the time? A diet that alters regular eating habits at all times, and for all time, while providing a balance in proteins, fats, starches, and even sugar, along with vitamins and minerals, is the only key to losing excessive weight and maintaining normal weight. Remember, doing this will in itself reduce high blood pressure proportionately, where overweight has been a predisposing factor.

It is usually unnecessary to restrict moderate use of salt or fluids, because of hypertension alone; a collateral medical condition may make the restriction necessary. Palatable substitutes for salt are available.

If you adhere strictly to the weight reducing diet, you should lose between 6 and 8 pounds a month. But the loss will not be along a straight downward diagonal line. You will reduce more and faster at the beginning of dieting. The reduction will be slower in later weeks and there will be periods of a week or longer in which, regardless of strict adherence to the diet, your weight will remain at a level, and may even increase slightly. Do not be upset by this; it is the normal response, caused by periodic retention of fluid which disappears abruptly, almost as mysteriously as it occurred, with a corresponding further loss in weight.

It is wise to keep a daily record of your weight. The best time to weigh yourself is in the morning immediately after arising.

Surgical Reduction

You may have heard that some obese persons, especially those who have a large "apron" of fat in the abdomen, submit to surgical operation to have the so-called apron removed. This is now rarely done. It is hazardous, healing is poor and it leaves an ugly scar. The only time that such an operation might be justified is when the apron of the fat is uncomfortable or causes severe skin irritation that does not clear up by any other treatment.

A new surgical method for fat reduction was described at the 1971 Annual meeting of the American Medical Association in Atlantic City. It is called a *gastroplasty*. Its use has not been long enough for a reliable evaluation but appears applicable only for the grossly overweight: persons weighing 350 pounds or more. Unless you weigh that much (and probably even if you do), my advice is to forget it; instead push away from the table.

Exercise

Exercise has always had popular appeal as a means of losing weight. Men and women with a few mild symptoms of hypertension, and moderate elevation of blood pressure as shown by the readings of the sphygmomanometer, may indulge in, and perhaps benefit from, moderate exercise: golfing, walking, riding, swimming, fishing, and not too violent dancing. Competitive sports are unwise because, in the heat of the game, you may not notice that you are overreaching yourself. You may climb stairs as long as it does not cause shortness of breath, chest pain, or undue fatigue. On this point, your doctor must advise you.

Do not deceive yourself that if you walk a lot, you will lose hundreds of calories and will have earned the right to eat beyond your allowed diet. Keep in mind that exercise also stimulates appetite.

Energy used up in walking about 2 miles equals 100 calories—a mere trifle. An adult must walk 36 miles at average speed to lose one pound of fat tissue. Loss is greater in hard physical labor. I have known golfers to lose 2 to 4 pounds and more after two rounds of golf on hot days. But this is due to loss of water while sweating and breathing. The loss is quickly regained by drinking fluids after the game. How practical is it to attempt significant reduction in weight by exercise alone? Exercise alone is of little value unless it is accompanied by reduction in food intake. Furthermore, exercise must be kept within the physical capacity of the person, according to his condition.

Steam Baths

Steam baths, sweat cabinets, and other fancy forms of hot baths will bring down your weight; but the loss is almost entirely due to loss of water. You will regain it immediately. If your heart is not in good order, steam baths, sauna baths, and such attempts at losing weight may not only be useless but actually dangerous.

I have said a great deal about weight and given the topic so much space because it is at the top of the list of what you can do to help yourself lower your blood pressure and at the same time reap beneficial side effects.

CHAPTER 10

COMPLICATIONS OF ESSENTIAL HIGH BLOOD PRESSURE

Complications are not likely for many years after high blood pressure is first detected. Complications are a late occurrence and do not always depend on how high your blood pressure is or for how long you have had it. As I have said many times before, the determining factor is the *condition of your arteries*. That generally means whether arteriosclerosis (hardening of the arteries) has developed. Almost all complications are caused by arteriosclerosis. Hypertension alone contributes mostly as a predisposing factor when it is not maintained under acceptable control.

Normally, the channels of arteries are lined by a smooth thin layer called the *intima* (Figure 4). In arteriosclerosis the intima becomes thicker as a result of formation of fibrous tissue and deposits of other substances, chiefly cholesterol, about which you have read and heard a great deal (Figure 5). Other fats may also be deposited. We do know that on examination of arteries at autopsy, arteriosclerotic arteries show such cholesterol deposits. The surface of the intima becomes rough, lumpy, cracked, and sometimes ulcerated. Thickening of the intima narrows the arterial channels and thus impedes the flow of blood. In addition, the abnormal surface of the intima favors the formation of clots, which in turn can further obstruct, even block, the flow of blood in the arteries.

The tissues and organs normally supplied by such arteries are then deprived of adequate blood carrying oxygen

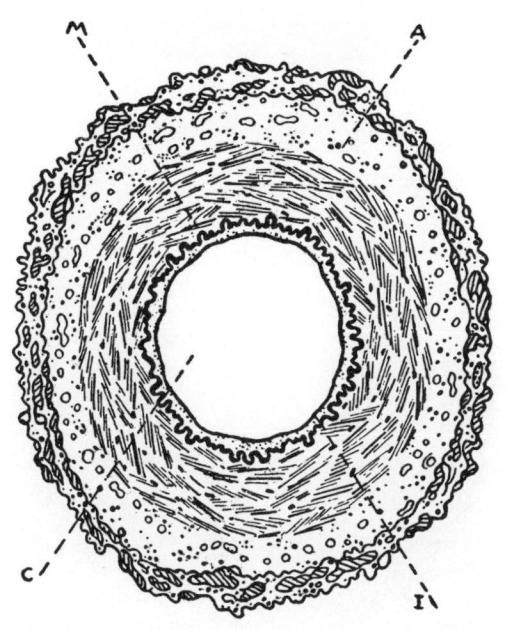

FIGURE 4. *Cross section of an artery.* The inner layer or intima (I) lines the channel (C). It is very smooth but is thrown up into small folds to permit distention of the artery when blood is pumped into it. The middle layer or media (M) is thick and is composed of elastic and muscular fibers which encircle the artery. The elastic fibers permit distention but limit its degree. The muscle fibers, when they contract, constrict the channel of the artery. The outer layer, or adventitia (A), is composed of strong fibrous tissue which reinforces the artery.

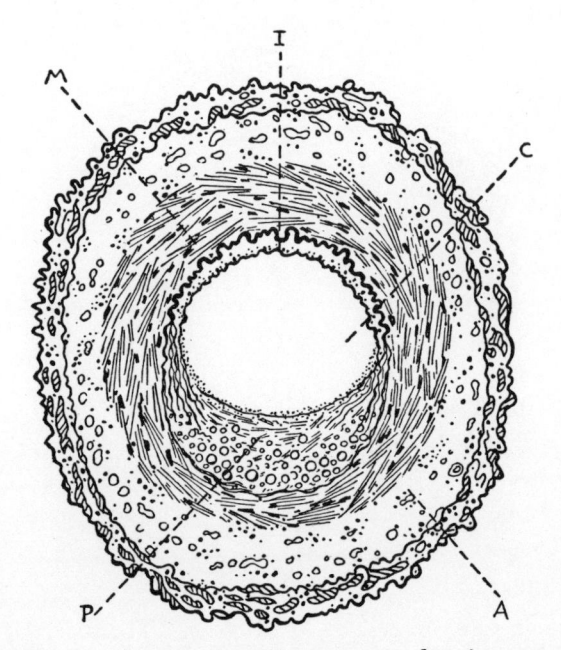

FIGURE 5. *Cross section of an artery showing arteriosclerosis (hardening).* The three layers are labeled as in figure 4. Note the deposit or plaque (P) on the intima which narrows the channel. The plaque is hard and its surface is rough.

and nutrients with the result that the tissues and organs become damaged and their functioning is impaired.

Your Heart

It is now well known that only about 10% of men and women with essential hypertension may eventually have serious kidney complications. This is far less than the possibility of an eventual heart attack or a stroke. Your heart, in fact, bears the brunt of complications. It is affected in about 60% to 75% of patients who have high blood pressure that has not been controlled and maintained. Let us trace the course of events and see why this is so. How the blood circulates and why the pressure goes up were discussed rather fully in Chapter 3. For those who may have skipped that chapter, some review may be helpful:

Blood leaves the heart by way of the aorta, a tube about 1¼ inches in diameter. Shortly after its origin, it divides into branches. In turn these branches continue to divide and subdivide to spread out to all parts of the body. Thus blood is distributed to every cell in the body. The very ends of the last branches, called arterioles (little arteries), have walls containing a relatively thick layer of muscular tissue which can contract and relax. The bore of their channels is so narrow that it is hard to imagine. When the muscular layer contracts, the channel becomes still narrower.

It should not be difficult to understand that widespread constriction of the channels impedes the flow of blood. But endlessly, the persistent heart keeps on pumping blood into arteries in normal amounts. The inevitable result is an increase in pressure exerted on the walls of the entire arterial system. The pressure backs up, so to speak, forcing the heart to pump harder in order to deliver a normal supply of blood to all parts of the body. That increased work on the part of the heart keeps up day and night. This, we believe, is what happens when your heart has to overcome high blood pressure. You know by now that high blood pressure favors the development of arteriosclerosis. Just why it does is not clear; but it does. When this change takes place in the *coronary arteries of the heart*, the heart begins to falter and symptoms develop.

The earliest change is *enlargement* of the heart, because its muscular component becomes thicker and increases in bulk, as do the biceps muscles of a prize fighter or the leg muscles of a professional dancer. The arteries of the heart do not increase their number or size to nourish the additional muscle bulk of the enlarged heart. The work must go on; but the blood supply with its oxygen and nutrients is no longer sufficient. In short, the overworked heart is on a reduced ration. It tries to continue as long as it can but eventually its capacity to perform the required work weakens until it becomes sick.

The Failing Pump

As I have said, the heart is composed almost entirely of muscle tissue (meat). Muscle tissue can contract, causing the heart to expel its contents. Then it relaxes and permits blood to enter the heart again. That is how the heart acts as a pump. It is likely that the heart could hold out for a longer time if it had to deal only with elevated blood pressure. Eventually, as I have emphasized here, high blood pressure favors the development of arteriosclerosis. This affects the heart's *coronary arteries* (crowning the heart but not a part of the circulatory system) as well as other arteries. The channels of the coronary arteries (which you have undoubtedly heard and read so much about) become narrower, and the blood supply to the heart muscle is further reduced. The heart is then unable to "take it" any longer, pumping becomes inefficient, and other heart disorders appear.

The symptoms produced by deficient pumping action

may begin with shortness of breath on exertion, climbing stairs at home, walking up a ramp to your seat at a football game, or walking anywhere for several blocks. Endurance becomes less and weakness begins to be felt more. Later the shortness of breath becomes more evident. It awakens you at night when you are asleep in your bed. You discover that you get relief by sitting up or by increasing the number of pillows. In more advanced forms, you may experience an attack such as that described on page 3.

Should shortness of breath be a symptom, do not wait for the entire drama to unfold. When you mention to your husband or wife how tired you get in the afternoon, that you can hardly drag yourself, your legs become heavy and your breathing a bit faster, do not brush off the advice to see your doctor, protesting that you know you need more sleep or a good workout at a gymnasium. Go at once to your doctor.

Your doctor finds your blood pressure is too high, your heart is somewhat enlarged, a new murmur is present, and, when he presses his fingertip firmly on the lower part of your leg, a definite depression remains. He hears clicking sounds in your lungs, evidence of congestion. The doctor tells you that your heart has weakened and recommends that you enter a hospital. You would be wise to agree.

Angina Pectoris

This is another heart complication which may develop in a patient who has hypertension. It is also a consequence of coronary arteriosclerosis with partial or complete obstruction in one of the branches. *Pain* in the chest is the outstanding symptom. It is frequently associated with a *feeling of tightness* or *constriction,* and *fear.* The pain and distress are generally located under the breastbone or across the upper part of the chest, and often spreads down one or both arms. The symptoms usually occur on walking, especially after a meal or an excitement. They cause the patient to stop in his tracks. The entire episode lasts only a few minutes and clears up when the patient stands or sits still. If he has been under treatment and has had nitroglycerine pills prescribed for him (which he always carries with him), the symptoms will usually clear in a few minutes when he places the small pill under his tongue.*

Coronary Thrombosis

This condition is becoming well known through all news media and exchange of experiences between friends. It is still better known as a heart attack. It is a third complication to which hypertensive persons are subject. Coronary thrombosis is caused by formation of a clot in a previously abnormal coronary artery, usually one affected by arteriosclerosis. The region of heart muscle formerly supplied by the affected artery is damaged and its functioning becomes impaired.

The onset of symptoms is generally abrupt. Pain resembling that in angina pectoris is typical but lasts hours or a few days as the dominant symptom. It may come on during activity, rest, or sleep. The appearance of the patient is often striking. His face becomes ashen gray, drops of sweat break out on his forehead, and he looks and feels exhausted. Weeks are required for recovery, and months for complete convalescence.*

Strokes

A stroke is damage to the brain caused by interference with or blocking of the arteries supplying the brain with blood. Another type of stroke is caused by bleeding (hemorrhage) into the substance of the brain.

How the Blood, Enriched with Oxygen and Nutrients,

─────────
* For further information, see my book: MANAGING YOUR CORONARY, published by Arco Publishing Company, Inc.

Reaches the Brain: Blood is carried to the brain by four arteries, two on each side of the neck. They course upward to the base of the skull where they pass through openings to enter the head. Once inside, the arteries branch and re-branch several times as they spread over the surface of the brain. From there, they send many small branches into the brain substance.

There are extensive connections between branches of the four arteries as they proceed upward along the sides of the neck and within the skull before they actually penetrate the brain. This meeting of the branches from one artery with the branches of another is called the *collateral circulation*. Its importance will be appreciated shortly. There is no significant joining between the vessels after they enter the brain proper.

Connections between the branches of the four arteries can limit damage to the brain, and even prevent it entirely, when a supplying artery is partly or completely obstructed. This is accomplished through by-passing the blood in the obstructed artery by way of the collateral circulation—the connecting branches of an obstructed and nearby unobstructed vessel. A glance at the accompanying schematic drawing of the collateral circulation will explain how the by-passing is accomplished (Figure 6).

Obstructive Strokes: The obstructive stroke is the common type. (Formerly we believed that bleeding into the brain was more frequent.) Obstructive strokes are the result of narrowing of the arterial channels in arteriosclerosis, or of obstruction from clot formation having the same underlying cause. Less frequently, small clots are carried by the blood stream from elsewhere in the body to the arteries supplying the brain. When the hardening process of arteriosclerosis sets in, in the arteries supplying blood to the brain, it makes itself known gradually by mild symptoms that at first attract little notice. If you were married

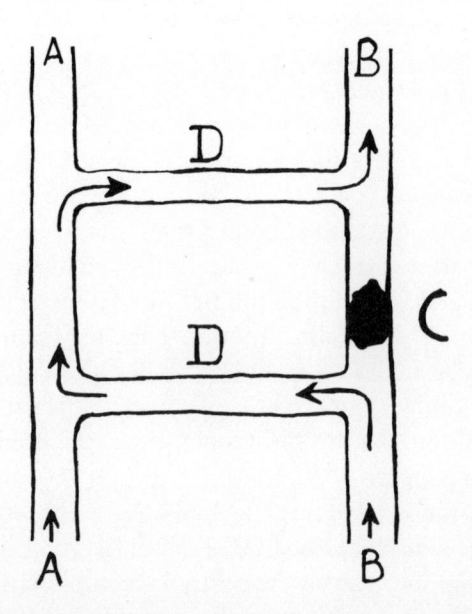

FIGURE 6. *Collateral circulation.* Schematic sketch: A and B are two arteries near each other in the neck. Blood flows upward in both to the brain. A branch from A meets a branch from B to form an open communication between arteries A and B. A similar arrangement is present at a higher level. Both of these open communications are labeled D. Follow the arrows:

A clot forms in artery B at C, completely obstructing this vessel. Blood flows straight up in A to the brain. Blood begins to flow upward in B but is stopped by the clot at C, thus forced to turn left at lower D to enter A and flow upward to upper D. There it goes right to return to B and at that point, it turns left to continue its upward passage in A to the brain. Thus, the obstruction at C is completely bypassed. Both communicating D channels comprise the collateral circulation.

to an absent-minded professor who seemed to be getting a bit grouchy, you would think he was just out of sorts that day. But if the forgetfulness and irritability grew to greater proportions than ever before, coupled with other changes in personality, such as sleeplessness, headache complaints, or untidiness, then you would have not simply an exasperating, but a truly sick man on your hands. If this should happen to your husband, do not go into a rage. Go to a doctor with him. If this happens to your wife, go to a doctor with her.

If hardening of the arteries has gone on for some time and the circulation in the blood vessels has slowed down, or a clot may be clinging to a rough patch on the lining of the arterial channel and forming a roadblock which deprives some part of the brain of its life-sustaining nourishment, then the collateral circulation sketched in Figure 6 may step in if necessary. If you are lucky, the affected area in the brain is small and not too important. Even if that area in the brain is larger and normally has important functions to perform, if the collateral circulation takes over in time, you may suffer nothing worse than a few moments of dizziness, loss of consciousness or temporary loss of power to speak or move some parts of your body. Such premonitory symptoms may recur for days or months before a major attack strikes.

The onset of a major attack is usually rather sudden. The patient may fall because he became unconscious, or he may slump to the ground because of paralysis of one of his legs. If the onset is during sleep, he may fall to the floor on attempting to get out of bed. Loss of consciousness may last only a few minutes, or as long as several hours, and during such episodes, the breathing becomes labored. Many patients nevertheless recover from the first major attack of obstructive stroke.

The doctor will examine for evidence of paralysis. He

will look at the face to see whether it draws to one side. He will lift each arm and leg in turn and allow it to fall. If paralyzed, it will fall heavily. If not, it will sink gradually to the bed. The doctor will also listen with his stethoscope over the arteries in the neck on both sides. A harsh murmuring sound will be produced by hardened arteries or incomplete obstructions in the arterial channel.

A spinal test may be necessary. The patient sits on the side of the bed, or, if he cannot do so, he is placed on his side. The skin over the lower part of the spine is sterilized with an antiseptic solution and a local anesthetic is injected between vertebrae selected in advance. A hollow needle is then inserted in the anesthetized area and a small amount of fluid is withdrawn for examination. The procedure, when properly performed, causes little, if any, discomfort. The information thus gained helps in recognizing whether the stroke is obstructive or due to bleeding in the brain. That test will also disclose whether some other condition is mimicking the symptoms of a stroke.

Another test consists in injecting a solution in a neck artery which makes that artery, especially its channel, visible on an x-ray. It also makes visible other arteries serving the brain, even within the skull. This enables the doctor to distinguish whether an arterial channel is narrowed, partly or completely obstructed, or whether the stroke is due to brain hemorrhage.

Not until the doctor has gained all the information that he needs can he plan treatment. Treatment may be medical with good nursing care and subsequent rehabilitation, or surgical removal of an obstruction in certain patients.

Stroke Caused by Bleeding: In strokes caused by bleeding, the cause is usually the bursting of an artery within the brain. Such burst arteries are usually arteriosclerotic and brittle, and the high blood pressure contributes to precipitating the accident.

The symptoms resemble those encountered in obstructive strokes except for some distinguishing signs: the onset is generally more abrupt and severe, loss of consciousness is deeper and more prolonged, and the spinal fluid contains evidence of bleeding. The distinctions, however, are less important than one might think. Treatment is about the same as in the obstructive type, but the outlook is generally not as favorable.

Needless Fear

Some people with high blood pressure live in fear of a stroke. Doctors try to make them see that strokes are not so common after all, and that if they do occur, the chances of survival and recovery are now in their favor. Like a great many human afflictions, this one has a worse reputation than it deserves. Try not to dwell on unhappy *possibilities*. Having a stroke is not a *probability*. Fear is bad for you. It does not stop anything, but it does raise your blood pressure. Think about immediate circumstances, immediate duties, immediate requirements, immediate care of personal and family health, immediate pleasures. Behave constructively and sensibly without dwelling uselessly on a vague future that is impossible to anticipate.

Let me tell you as convincingly as I can that serious symptoms, such as persistent or severe headaches, dizziness or tingling, pain or numbness in your limbs, fingers, or toes need not be the heralds of a stroke. You can talk yourself into believing that headaches as bad as yours must be a sign of some fearful fate awaiting you. The positive action is to see your doctor and find out what the situation is. The severity of symptoms seems individual. Some exaggerate every discomfort and make it the sole subject of conversation. Some ignore symptoms, which is equally foolish. See about them where something can be done about them, where their meaning can be understood, namely at a doctor's office or clinic. A headache or other symptom need not mean excessively high blood pressure or advanced hardening of the arteries. If they did, worrying about the symptoms and talking about them with relatives and neighbors and anyone who will listen will only make you a bore while you neglect the one sensible move: to see your doctor, find out, take his reassurance, and follow his instructions. We can say only that some men and women have violent symptoms; others get off more lightly. Aggravated symptoms do not always mean aggravated hypertension. Take my words as sincere advice to take care of hypertension but to forget about strokes.

On the other hand, if you or someone close to you should by chance have a stroke, then, again, hold fast to the hopeful aspects. The degree of injury and the extent of brain damage determine the outcome. Many recover completely; others recover within useful limits. Remarkable orthopedic devices are now available to help rehabilitation. To be greatly disabled as a result of a stroke is now exceptional.

Rehabilitation centers and medicine have changed the outlook for people who have had strokes, just as it has for those who had poliomyelitis or other disabling conditions. They can get about, perform serviceable work, support themselves, and pursue any interest. And most of them do.

CHAPTER 11

SECONDARY HYPERTENSION: SYMPTOM OF UNDERLYING AILMENT

Reader, you will recall that I mentioned that hypertension is of two types (page 23): essential hypertension, about which everything that has preceded has referred, and secondary hypertension, in which case the high blood pressure is a symptom of another disease, an underlying illness. That illness can be detected and recognized, and if it can be eradicated, as it often can, then the high blood pressure will be lowered, and the pressure will return to normal or near normal reading.

Incomplete Constriction of the Great Artery

You know by now that the great artery running from the heart is the aorta. It takes purified blood out to all parts of the body. It may be hampered in its work by a defect called *coarctation* which means *constriction*. In *coarctation of the aorta* (which is the technical designation of the title of this topic: *Incomplete Constriction of the Great Artery*) there is a form of hypertension in which the blood pressure in the upper part of the body is extremely high while in the lower part, the legs, for example, it is lower than normal. Both the high blood pressure in the upper part of the body and the low pressure in the lower part can be corrected by a relatively safe surgical operation.

Shortly after the juncture of the aorta and the heart,

arteries run out from the aorta to take blood to the arms, head, and neck. Farther away from your heart, the aorta divides and gives off branches leading to lower parts of the body, including the legs. In some people there is a narrowing or incomplete constriction, a coarctation, of the section of the aorta just beyond the branch to the left arm, but before the branches to the lower part of the body are given off. Its effect is to impede the flow of blood to the lower parts of the body; for while the blood flows properly in your upper parts, it cannot pass so easily through the narrowed part of the aorta. Since your heart continues to drive blood into the aorta as if all were well, the pressure rises above the roadblock and falls beyond it. That isn't hard to follow, is it? Just picture when something blocks traffic on a two-way highway leading to a sudden bridge where the road narrows to a single lane. Blood pressure rising in the aorta and its branches between the heart and the narrowed segment may reach over 200 systolic and the diastolic may still remain unchanged or may reach to about 120 in the upper part of your body. Meanwhile, beyond the roadblock, the systolic blood pressure becomes drastically reduced as does the diastolic. This is registered in your lower trunk and legs. The story of a young patient and how this trouble was corrected will illustrate coarctation of the aorta:

A 17-year-old high school student was put through a routine medical examination just after school had started in the fall. The girl had had headaches, her feet were always cold, and she felt tired most of the time. Her systolic blood pressure was 205 and her diastolic, 107, both far too high. The doctor tried to take her pulse in the thigh, back of the knee, and at the ankles. There was none, which immediately suggested to him coarctation of the aorta. Special x-rays showed the telltale notchings at the lower margins of some ribs, and a side view of her chest disclosed a localized narrowing of the aorta in the expected location. Finding x-ray confirmation of the coarctation explained the patient's symptoms. The headaches were caused by the very high blood pressure within the arteries in her head, her feet and legs were cold because of lowered blood flow in the arteries in the lower part of her body and legs, and her weakness was caused by inadequate blood supply to the muscles in that area.

Before 1945 patients with coarctation of the aorta could not expect to live more than half the normal life span. A solution was not available. Now we correct the defect in the aorta by a surgical procedure in which the narrowed segment is resected and the ends of the aorta are brought close together and stitched. If a larger section of the aorta must be removed, so large that it cannot be brought together, a graft is implanted to replace the resected part.

It is an exciting but not a particularly dangerous operation. More than 95% survive without difficulty, a rate of 1% or 2% more than any other major surgical operation. The results are excellent and many thousands of such operations have now been performed successfully all over the world.

Nephritis

Hypertension is an important symptom of nephritis, a form of kidney disease. Our knowledge concerning nephritis, its cause, its cure, and other aspects—is still far from complete, although it has been studied intensely by scientists since it was first described nearly 150 years ago.

In 1934, Dr. Harry Goldblatt, a Cleveland physician, discovered an experimental way to produce long-standing high blood pressure in animals. He learned that reducing the blood supply to the kidneys can cause high blood pressure. His further experiments demonstrated that, if the blood supply is cut down even further than he had done at first, the blood pressure rises still more. There comes a point at which the impaired kidneys manufacture a substance named *angiotonin*, meaning something causing tone in the blood vessels. When he injected angiotonin into other dogs but left their kidneys alone, hypertension developed. The angiotonin's effect was directly on the smallest vessels—the arterioles—constricting them and reducing their diameter (see page 97). When angiotonin is injected into a volunteer person whose blood pressure is normal, the pressure rises within a few minutes. It passes off almost immediately, however; harm is not done. We know that the blood supply of human kidneys sometimes flows through severely narrowed arteries and arterioles. Illuminating to science are the hypertensive patients with one sound and one damaged kidney. Researchers reasoned that if the kidney whose blood supply has become limited and now manufactures angiotonin were removed, the patient would be rid of hypertension. That is exactly what happens. (The problem of hypertension, however, still awaits complete solution.)

Uremia: Uremia develops mostly when kidney function is greatly impaired or entirely lost. It is usually the result of severe kidney disease. The kidneys are then unable to excrete toxic waste substances collected by the blood. The toxic substances accumulate in the blood and are then distributed throughout the body in concentrated form, sufficient to cause severe and widespread damage throughout the body. When that happens, the patient dies of uremia.

A case in point is that of a lonely person who was found by a maid during her regular rounds in the rooming house where the woman lived. Information was not available about her. Her breathing was labored: rapid and deep, and her breath had an ammonia-like odor, somewhat like that of urine. Her lungs were congested; her systolic blood pressure was 214 and her diastolic, 117. (These terms are familiar to you now; if not, see page 15.) These were valuable clues. Did she have uremic poisoning?

While blood was being drawn from a vein in the arm for chemical tests for uremia, diabetic coma, overdose of insulin, or overdose of sleeping pills, a catheter (a rubber tube) was inserted into her bladder to obtain urine. Examination of the urine took less time than other tests and could be helpful in detecting most of the conditions causing stupor. But the bladder was empty. The kidneys had not been producing any urine and there was no way of telling how long this had been the situation. The patient's condition was becoming worse; every minute counted.

The first report from the chemistry laboratory indicated that the blood showed evidence of severe uremia. It was essential to find the cause of the uremia; the kind of treatment depended on that information. The common causes of uremia are Bright's disease (or nephritis) as discussed on page 71. In some other conditions the onset of uremia is usually more gradual. Here it was obviously abrupt and overwhelming. In bygone days, doctors would have been at a loss for further efforts to save the patient. Not so now. An *intravenous pyelogram* was performed. In this procedure, a solution of a special form of iodine is injected into a vein (*intravenous*) near the bend of the elbow. After a short time the iodine solution collects inside the kidneys. The solution is there concentrated by the kidneys within a few minutes, making the kidneys and their inside opaque, so that their size, shape, inside, and concentrating ability casts a shadow on an x-ray film. This picture we call a *pyelogram*. The results were not satisfactory, however, and more valuable time had been lost.

One more test was left to try: an x-ray procedure disclosing the condition of the arteries that supply blood to the kidneys, showing especially the condition of the arterial channels. Those x-ray films showed that the arteries supplying blood to both kidneys were almost completely occluded, closed. That represented a desperate situation. If the blood circulation could not be restored quickly, the kidneys would degenerate beyond recovery; uremia would get worse rapidly, and the patient would die.

A competent vascular surgeon (an expert on arteries and veins) was in the hospital at the time. His opinion was that her only chance was by an immediate operation to reopen the channels of the arteries to restore blood supply to both kidneys. After a time, the surgeon looked up and, although most of his face was covered by the surgical mask, a smile was evident. The operation was successful. While in the recovery room under close observation for the next 14 hours, the patient passed more than a quart of urine. The next day, it was two quarts, and from then on the patient who almost died of uremia improved rapidly. From a medical standpoint, we are fortunate to be living in the present age.

Laymen often connect high blood pressure with fatal kidney disorders. However, doctors learned only a few years back that this belief is not true and that our job is to bring the public over to the newer point of view.

Kidney complications, when and if they occur, enter late—many years late in the drama of hypertension. The blood pressure may become exceedingly high, often over 230 systolic, but that in itself is not a great threat. Many patients go on for years with such pressures. Headaches are common and the kidneys begin to function imperfectly. Waste products and toxic substances (normally carried by the blood to the kidneys to be excreted in the urine) are not thrown off as well as under normal conditions. As a result, they accumulate in the blood and produce symptoms.

Treatment resolves itself into a diet containing less than usual amounts of salt. Completely salt-free diets are not widely ordered, because they are monotonous and may add to the discomfort that the patient already endures. The heart may need support if it begins to falter, but your doctor will take care of that as well as the salt content indicated by your diet.

Reduction of high blood pressure is important; but, unless the reason to reduce it rapidly is urgent, it must be accomplished gradually and cautiously. Powerful medicines in fairly large doses may cause an abrupt or rapid drop in blood pressure which may further impair kidney function. Or, undesired effects may be produced on the heart or brain. It is not at all rare to cause transient faintness or momentary loss of consciousness by too aggressive treatment causing too abrupt and too great a drop in blood pressure.

Surgical procedures by which the sympathetic nerves were cut to reduce high blood pressure have been almost abandoned.

The Great Breakthrough

Of all the complications that can afflict patients with high blood pressure, those affecting the kidneys are the most serious. Nowadays, however, *dialysis* with the aid of the artificial kidney and dialysis by way of the peritoneum (the lining within the abdomen) have changed the outlook from one of hopelessness to one of hope. *Dialysis* is the scientific term for the things that happen when two solutions are separated by a porous membrane, like cellophane. In addition, transplantation of kidneys has proved practical and lifesaving. These new methods of treatment have revolutionized our concepts of kidney disorders and how to treat them effectively, including when they are complications of high blood pressure (Figures 7, 8, 9, and 10).

The Artificial Kidney: Take a piece of cellophane or cuprophane, make it into a bag, and fill it with water. It will not leak. Yet, when magnified thousands of times, you

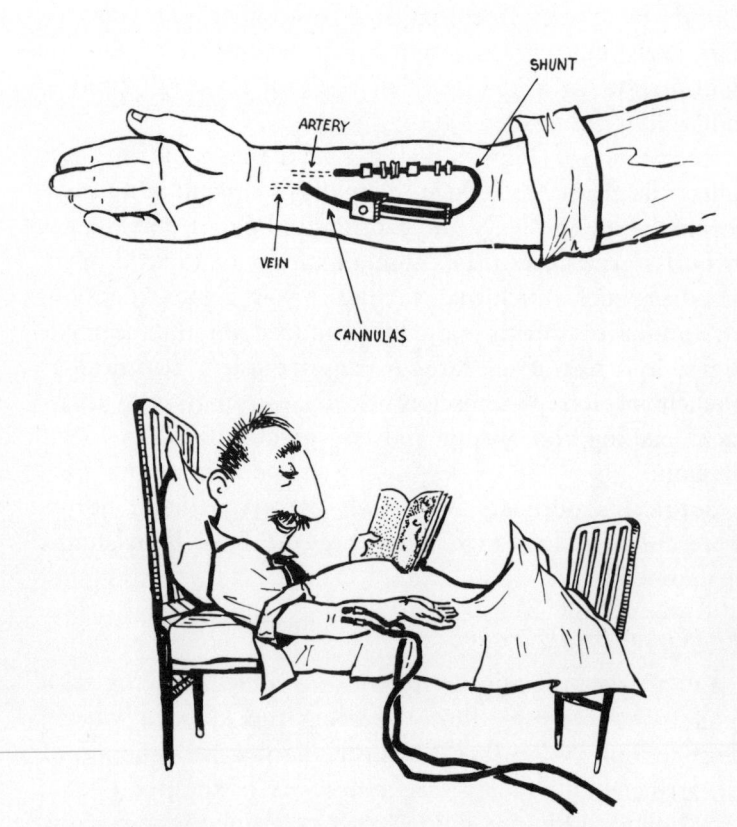

FIGURE 7. *Long-standing dialysis via blood vessels in the arm or leg.* Upper Figure: Two tiny plastic tubes, the cannulas, are used. One is inserted in an artery, the other, in a vein. Their protruded ends are connected by a shunt which permits blood flow from one cannula to the other between treatments.

Lower Figure: At the time of treatment, the shunt is removed and the cannulas are connected to tubes leading to the artificial kidney machine. There the blood is cleansed and returned to the patient. The patient can read, sleep or visit with other patients while the cleansing is going on. See text for more details.

would see that sheets of these materials have millions of tiny holes, called pores. Cellophane and cuprophane are the basic parts of an amazing device called an *artificial kidney*. The artificial kidney is a rather large machine containing sheets of the materials mentioned. Blood from the patient passes between such sheets to be purified by the process called *dialysis*.

You can gain a good idea of what happens by performing a simple experiment:

Make a solution of salt by putting some in a cellophane bag full of pure water. Seal it. Place the bag of salt solution in a container of pure water. Soon the pure water in the container will become salty, while the salt solution in the bag will lose strength. Eventually there will be salt solution of equal strength in the container and in the cellophane bag. This takes place because the dissolved particles of salt are small enough to pass through the pores in the cellophane bag. Although particles pass through the cellophane *in both directions, more pass from the stronger to the weaker solution* when each differs in strength. The process by which particles pass through the cellophane membrane is called *dialysis*.

Normally, waste products, water, toxic and other unnecessary substances are collected by the circulating blood from all parts of the body, as explained in Chapter 3. The blood carries the waste products to the kidneys where they are excreted in the form of urine. But when in the late stages of high blood pressure, kidney function becomes impaired, the kidneys can no longer excrete the waste from the body. As a result they accumulate in the blood and cause serious consequences. Uremic poisoning is one of the most serious of these consequences.

The artificial kidney is now available to remove the undesirable substances from the blood and regulates the amount of water in the body by dialysis. This process

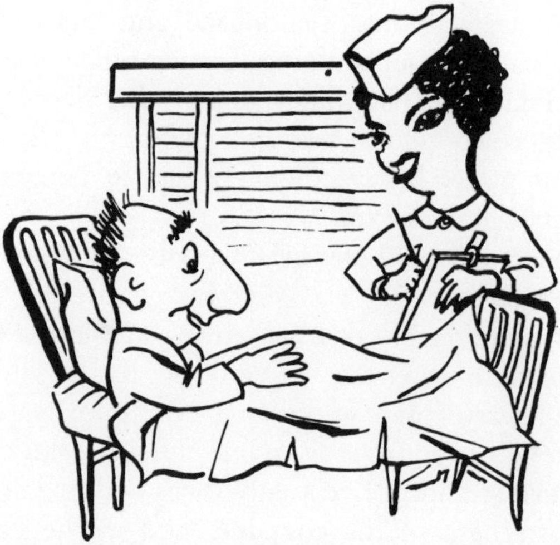

FIGURE 8. *Where the patient can be dialyzed.* Dialysis may be performed in a dialysis center, usually in a hospital. It can be done at home after the patient learns how.

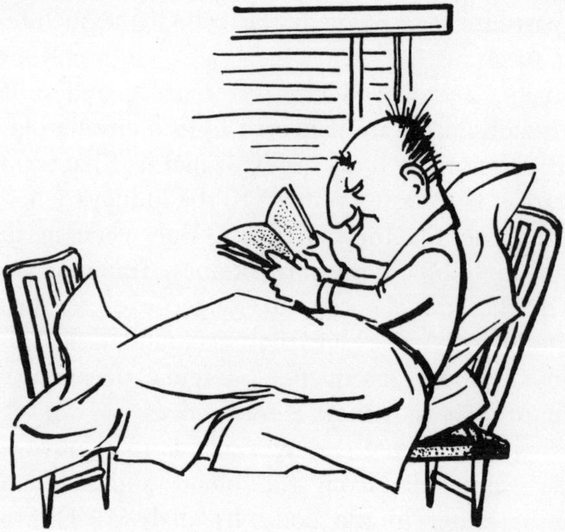

diminishes or removes the danger and gives the kidneys a chance to rest and recover. In the artificial kidney, a cellophane sheet is located between compartments containing blood from the patient and a cleansing fluid called the *dialysate*. Recall the experiment of the salt water in a cellophane bag placed in a container of pure water. In the same way, any dissolved particles in the blood or dialysate, small enough to pass through the pores, will do so. They pass back and forth in both directions. Many unwanted substances dissolved in the blood may also be dissolved in the dialysate. Dialysate is free of body waste; thus, these particles pass out into the cleansing fluid and can be discarded. The blood may have become deficient in certain essential chemical substances during uremia. If these needed substances are added to the dialysate, they, too, will pass into the blood during dialysis.

Dialysis treatments are given about three times a week, each session lasting about 6 hours. This is best done in a hospital. The patient lies on a cot or bed while he is connected to the artificial kidney machine by which his blood receives a thorough bath, so to speak. Treatments are continued until the patient's blood and general condition return as close as possible to a normal state. During treatments patients are comfortable; they may do whatever they like—read, converse, or listen to stock market reports or music.

Another type of blood dialysis is less confining. Patients who undergo it may attend to their affairs except for a visit to a treatment center about once a week. In the intervals between treatments, the patient is at home and goes to work, carrying on normal activities. In this type of dialysis, thin plastic tubes are placed in an arm or leg. The protruding ends of the tubes are connected by a shunt tube, permitting blood to flow from one tube into the other between treatments. When a treatment is to be given, the

118   SECONDARY HYPERTENSION

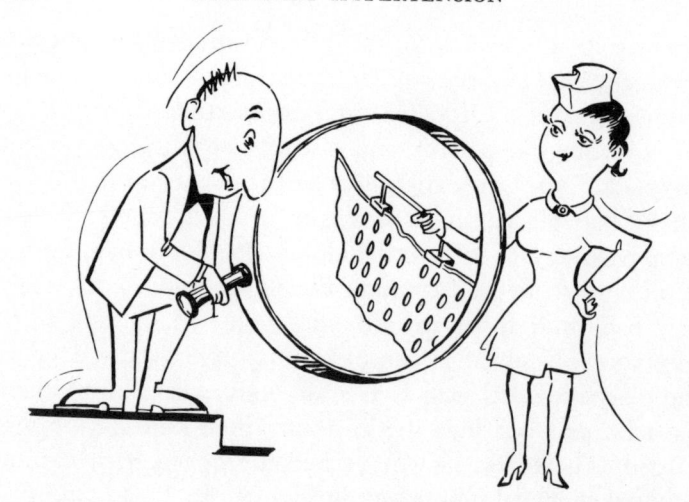

FIGURE 9. *How dialysis works.* Make a cellophane bag. Fill it with water. Does it leak? No. It is full of holes. Cellophane has millions of tiny holes. Magnified thousands of times, cellophane looks like either one of these. Cellophane is the basic part of the artificial kidney. This explanation is in the text.

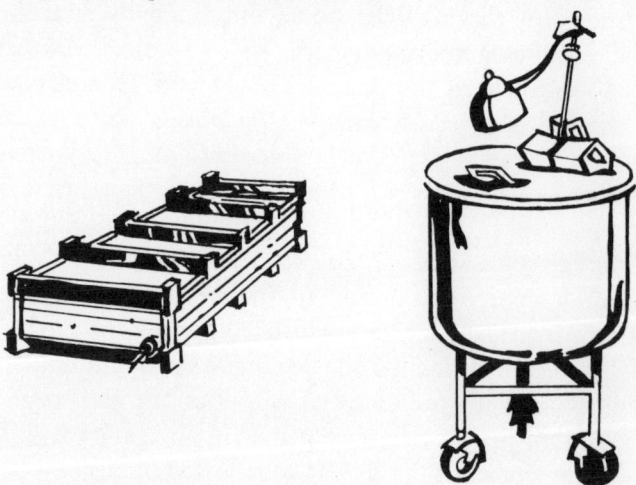

FIGURE 10. *Two models showing how the artificial kidney looks from the outside.*

shunt tube is removed and the tubes in the artery and vein are connected to an artificial kidney machine for purifying. During treatments the patient is relaxed; he can read, sleep, or visit with friends, and all the while his blood is being cleansed. Afterward the shunt is replaced and he can leave until the next scheduled treatment.

Abdominal (Peritoneal) Dialysis: A third type of dialysis is a simpler procedure than the method just described, but it is best suited for short-term dialysis. Abdominal pain is possible in the early stages of this type of dialysis. It is about a fifth as effective as the method just described. The method first described is preferred when dialysis must be repeated or maintained for a long time.

Inside the abdomen is a lining, a thin layer or membrane, which can act in a manner similar to the cellophane described.

Local anesthesia is induced in a small area in the midline of the abdomen about an inch below the navel. A thin tube is pushed through the anesthetized area until it reaches the lower left part of the abdomen. The other end of the tube is connected to bottles of dialysate, the cleansing agent. About 2 quarts of warmed dialysate are run into the abdominal cavity and allowed to remain for about 30 minutes before being drained. The thin tube is pulled out, but may be reinserted later if necessary.

The use of dialysis as an effective method for treating serious kidney disorders must be considered a major scientific breakthrough, the equal of any discovered in recent years.

Transplantation of Kidneys: Dialysis and transplantation are today the established treatments for kidney damage formerly considered hopeless. The transplantation of kidneys from one person to another is an even greater achievement than dialysis. Transplantation is preferable because of the limitations that any type of dialysis imposes on the patient. With successful transplantation, patients can lead an almost normal life. Women with kidney transplants have had successful pregnancies.

The incidence of survival after transplantation keeps improving. In 1970 Dr. Starzl reported on a follow-up study of patients who received kidney transplants. The period of observation after operation varied from 2 years to 7½ years. There were 131 consecutive patients who received transplants from a member of the family. Of these, 91 were still living. Of 58 patients who received a kidney from an unrelated donor, only 19 were still living during this period of follow-up observation. The lesson is that *success of a transplanted kidney is likelier if the kidney is received from a member of the family*.

From another report we learn that frequent success was achieved in about 3,000 kidney transplants performed during the ten years from 1961 to 1971.

Surgical replacement of a kidney is not the obstacle. The technical aspects of such an operation are well within the capability of an experienced kidney surgeon. Of far greater importance now is how to prevent or successfully treat *rejection of the implanted kidney by the patient who receives it*. Rejection, of course, is involuntary. We have gained considerable information on preventing rejection and we have put it to use with the result that enormous progress has already been made, with every prospect of increasing success in overcoming the problem of rejection.

You know that the blood contains red cells and white cells. There are several kinds of white blood cells. Those in which we are interested here are the small *lymphocytes*. These are important in the rejection of a transplanted kidney. When a kidney is implanted in the recipient, the small lymphocytes normally present in the blood of the patient receiving the graft begin to infiltrate the implanted kidney to cause its rejection. Fortunately, this does not happen in every case, as you will learn shortly.

As you have read, it is easier to prevent rejection and have a good result than to attempt treatment. We now know that the most important single factor is proper selection of a kidney donor. If success is to be attained, the best chances for success in a kidney transplant can be attained when there is a similarity between donor and recipient. The hereditary factor in both donor and recipient must be as similar as possible. It is for this reason that two siblings having the same father and mother make the best match, with a near 90% chance for complete success for an indefinite but long period. A parent and his offspring also make a good transplantation match, but not as good as brothers and/or sisters. The outlook in an unrelated pair have the poorest chance, something like a 15% chance for success against rejection. With time and newer knowledge, this rate will surely improve. With time and newer knowledge, the breakthrough of overcoming the body's built-in habit of rejection of a foreign body (which a stranger's kidney tissue represents to the recipient's natural agents of rejection) will surely become a reality. Researchers are continually at work on the problem. When that day of reality comes, kidney transplants of unrelated donors will be as successful as those of related donors.

Pheochromocytoma

Another type of secondary hypertension is caused in 85% of the cases by a tumor in the adrenal glands, elsewhere in the abdomen in 10%, or in the chest or neck in about 5%. The tumor, called *pheochromocytoma*, is in most instances benign, which means that it does not recur when completely removed by operation.

These tumors manufacture large amounts of epinephrine and norepinephrine which get into the blood. Both of them are capable of causing *high blood pressure* and other symptoms. The rise in blood pressure is characteristically intermittent, but it may persist. Again, bear in mind that I am describing an underlying disease in which hypertension is secondary—one of several symptoms of the basic disorder. If you have the common variety of essential hypertension, pheochromocytoma need not concern you. But, you must find out what type of hypertension you have. The persistent form of pheochromocytoma produces severe symptoms easily mistaken for severe essential hypertension, including the complications of essential hypertension.

The intermittent attacks produce spells of hypertension which last from minutes to hours, reaching heights of 200 to 300 systolic. This is the dominant feature. During the spell, severe headaches, profuse sweating, and palpitation are experienced. Other symptoms are anxiety, trembling, rapid heart beat, pain in the region of the heart, the abdomen or back, nausea, vomiting, sugar in the urine, and pallor or flushing of the face.

It is important that the doctor recognize pheochromocytoma. This is a serious ailment; it can prove fatal. Mercifully, it is almost always cured by surgical operation. Fortunately a specific test is known for recognition of pheochromocytoma, so that the diagnosis can be assured and the operation performed. The test measures epinephrine and norepinephrine or their products as found in a 24-hour specimen of urine. When the presence of the tumor is known, the location of the tumor is found by x-ray examinations. Treatment, surgical removal of the tumor or tumors, is preferably done by an experienced surgeon. Cure with return of the blood pressure to normal or near normal can be expected within two or three days after a complete operation. This is because the hypertension was a symptom of this basic serious disease.

Primary Hyperaldosteronism (Rare)

Primary hyperaldosteronism is a *rare* cause of secondary hypertension. The ailment was first recognized in human beings in 1955, thus it is a fairly recent medical disclosure. It is characterized by two main features. First is the symptom of high blood pressure which is generally mild. However, it can lead to the more serious consequences of uncontrolled high blood pressure: enlargement of the heart, heart failure, headaches, and in this case, impairment of the eyes. The second feature is the excessive loss of potassium from the body. This results in extreme muscle weakness, paralysis, muscle cramps, and frequency of urination day and night. Potassium is abnormally low in the blood, but excessive in the urine; the blood potassium is lost in the urine.

Primary hyperaldosteronism can usually be cured or at least greatly relieved by slowly returning the blood pressure to normal values. This can be accomplished through surgical removal of a tumor of the adrenal gland, occasionally even if it is a cancerous tumor, or by removing part of the adrenal glands, if they contain too much tissue but a tumor is not present. The underlying cause of the hypertension is obviously the adrenal gland's disturbance.

The body cannot afford to lose too much potassium through urination. That is why when *diuretics* are prescribed, supplemental potassium is often prescribed to make up for the loss through urination. Fruits, particularly bananas, cantaloupe, and orange juice are also rich in potassium. An interesting current sidelight was the loss of potassium through prolonged weightlessness experienced by the astronauts of Apollo 15. The loss temporarily affected the beat of their hearts.

Cushing's Syndrome

A disturbed function of the adrenal gland was first recognized in 1932 by Dr. Harvey W. Cushing, an American brain surgeon. The disorder is known by his name.

In this rare condition the adrenal glands secrete too much

cortisone. Both adrenal glands are usually involved: the glands may contain too much or too active tissue (60%), a tumor (30%), less often, cancer. The adrenal glands may appear normal (10%). Some authorities believe that the pituitary gland, a gland located at the base of the skull, enters into the disturbance. Cushing's syndrome when it is observed, however rarely, is likely to be in women between 30 and 40 years of age.

The symptoms resemble those induced by long or excessive use of cortisone. The face, neck, and trunk are obese; the face appears bloated ("moon face"); a hump, called a camel's hump, develops high up on the back; irregular whitish stripes resembling scars appear on the abdomen. The other chief manifestations are weakness, shrinkage of the muscles, *high blood pressure* (but not as a lone symptom), hemorrhages into the skin causing purplish blotches, softening of the bones resulting in backache—a picture resembling diabetes and susceptibility to infection and fractures of the spine.

Successful surgical intervention can bring about significant improvement and regression of the high blood pressure, or make the ailment more amenable to medication.

I have mentioned this disease because it exists; but bear in mind that it is *rare*.

The Pill

Although there is really no connection, I cannot leave the subject of secondary hypertension without mentioning one more example that is closely linked to modern times: The Pill. A few women taking The Pill for contraceptive purposes have hypertension, requiring that The Pill be discontinued.

CHAPTER 12

LIVING WITH HIGH BLOOD PRESSURE: RULES FOR THE HYPERTENSIVE

In the light of what I hope you have learned through reading this book, to get the best out of the situation, you yourself must give your doctor intelligent support. I hope that I have helped you to understand something about how your body functions. It remains for you to follow your doctor's directions and to govern your daily life accordingly. No matter how brilliant a physician he may be, or how inspired the devices of science on which he draws, the successful effect on your health in the long run is largely in your own hands. For you and those close to you who have high blood pressure, these rules are a guide:

1. *See your doctor early*. If you have any reason to think that something is wrong, go to your doctor. It is not babyish to make an appointment and say, "I just don't feel well." He can probe with questions and find out where and how by the detailed examination described for you earlier. The sooner you go, the better chance he has of helping you. After the age of 40, have a medical checkup at least once a year whether or not you feel well.

2. *Do not diagnose yourself*. My explanations of the problems of diagnosis should have made plain to you that even to the expert, hypertension is not always easy to recognize until it has been measured. Your doctor will admit that he does not know all the answers, but he knows many of them and he can draw on experience to decide

what is best for you. Be grown up about it and admit that you may be a good businessman, a good housekeeper, a good decorator, or a good file clerk; but you are *not* a physician. Put your health in the hands of a physician in whom you have confidence and ignore the prescriptions of your friends. They are not physicians either. Ignore the sales pitches of TV, magazine and newspaper advertisements, written by advertising agencies' writers. In all probability they are not physicians, and in any case, they are acting salesmen first.

3. *Be moderate in all things.* That is an ancient Golden Rule. The Greek sage Solon said to overdo nothing. This is a good rule for both the sound and the sick. Work, play, and eat with zest—but not too hard. Avoid becoming overtired. Your symptoms: headaches, shortness of breath, dizziness, and disturbed vision are your absolute stop signs. When the signals go on, stop, look and listen. Stop what you are doing, take it easy, and be sure to tell your doctor what happened. Better still, don't let yourself reach this point. When you rest, your blood pressure goes down. Even extremely high pressure can be significantly brought down by days in bed. At one time, that was the best and almost the only help we could offer. Even if in the end, your blood pressure returns to its earlier high level, your arteries will have had at least that much relief. Fluctuating blood pressure is easier on your blood vessels and your organs than persistently high blood pressure.

4. A short nap or quiet half hour after luncheon can be beneficial, if you can possibly manage it.

5. Do not run up stairs.

6. Eat four or five light meals rather than three heavy ones.

7. One cup of coffee is better than two. You may have two if your doctor consents—but no more. If you are not a coffee drinker, do not begin now. If you are and the

so-called coffee break seems to relax you, then drink one of the readily available decaffeinated types on the market.

8. Smoke not more than three cigars a day or half a dozen cigarettes, or one or two pipefuls, if you are already a smoker and believe that you cannot quit. You can, if you will genuinely try. If you are not a smoker, do not begin now.

9. One glass of beer a day will not hurt you. Regarding other alcoholic drinks, consult your doctor.

10. Go to bed before midnight.

11. Take exercise, but again, in moderation. Avoid competitive strenuous sports unless you have the strength of mind to let sturdier fellows win; avoid competitive sports if your physical condition is not the best. Winning or even playing may cost *you* too much effort.

12. *Stick to suitable work*. Most hypertensive persons can continue their mode of life, making only those changes in diet and exercise that promote their general well-being. Some must make a change. This will be decided by the state of your health and by the nature of your customary work. If you and your doctor think it best to retire, ideally this may be done—if your health and money permit it— by easy stages, tapering the day's work gradually. When the time comes for complete withdrawal from active life, you should have prepared yourself for it mentally and by having cultivated hobbies, or better still, by devoting yourself to a good cause; there are so many of them. You will help yourself by helping others. It may sound like a trite saying, but it is so in this case only because it is true.

13. *Watch your weight*. Obesity is ugly, hampering, and dangerous. Life insurance companies over the years have compared the records of thousands of fat people with those of men and women of normal weight; the fat die young. Pound by pound, they shorten their expectation of life. If you want to live, reduce; you can do it.

14. *Cultivate a calm mind.* You must break the vicious circle of worrying because you have high blood pressure, and having high blood pressure because you worry. Worry raises your blood pressure, robs you of sleep, makes you miserable, and perhaps costs you your friends. Only you know what it is costing your husband or your wife or your children. When things go wrong, do your best and endure the rest. Help where you can; do what you must. No one's life is free from cares and anxieties. But if you keep calm, you can think straighter and do more. Some distress is inevitable for everyone, but realizing that your situation is not unique, that it is a part of living may help you to train yourself to a wholesome attitude.

15. *Make the most of your life.* Making the most of life does not mean squandering it. It means guarding it while enjoying what is permissible to you and available to you. Do not be afraid of your ailment. Be hopeful and try to forget yourself *after* you have done the constructive things suggested to you by your doctor, your good sense, I hope, and by me.

If you have always dedicated your life to getting ahead in our "cash culture," as so many hypertensive persons do, stop to ask yourself what it is costing you and whether it is worth it. Find some worthy and selfless interest. Take time from work to cultivate that interest. It will make you a more interesting and a healthier person. It is dismaying to encounter someone who is so immersed in his own money-making business that he cannot converse about anything else. It is equally disheartening to meet someone so introverted that he or she cannot think of anyone else beyond the amenities, and anything said serves only as a jumping-off point to discuss personal ailments.

A good place to start making the most of life is by taking time to enjoy one's own family, enjoying life with them, remembering an old friend too long neglected. So many worthy charities await volunteers to aid with time even if they cannot help with money. What happened to the little talents you tinkered with in your youth? How about trying your hand at them again?

I do not know what your inclinations are: art? writing? music? When was the last time you wrote someone a really good letter, one that would gladden the heart? When was the last time you read a really good book, better still, reread one that you always liked and meant to read again? When was the last time you enjoyed the envelopment of a room full of inspired painting or sculpture, in a museum you have meant to visit? When have you listened quietly to music? What are you waiting for? How are you at growing plants? Finally and again, a hypertensive person can find satisfaction and serenity in giving of himself or herself to a clinic, a hospital, a rest home, or such an organization as the American Heart Association, about which I have reminded you. Science needs all the moral and financial backing it can get—and a little more time to bring to light the cause of hypertension, and its sure cure. You do not need to be a scientist to give that help, just a good person who can extend thinking outside one's own body.

Chapter 13

The Promise of Science

You may reasonably ask why, if your body is so adaptable to changing conditions, your blood pressure does not retreat within proper bounds instead of staying too high. That question, as I said at the beginning, we cannot yet answer. Before instruments for measuring were available, we barely understood that high blood pressure was a reality; consequently we could not diagnose the condition. Now we know that most cases are due to spasm or narrowing of the arterioles, the smallest arteries. But this is not the complete story. What causes the spasm and narrowing of the arterioles? We have some answers, as indicated throughout this book, but not all the answers.

Diagnosis was and is the first step toward correcting the difficulty, this we are able to achieve. We have learned how to control the condition and what makes it worse and improves it. We have still to take the next step, the discovery of the absolute cause. Once we have gone that far, the final step, the *cure*, may be comparatively simple. In the meantime, we must wait; but we may wait with hope, because all over the nation, in the hospitals, universities, research centers, and the commercial pharmaceutical laboratories, some of the best trained minds in the country are working hard to unlock the last mystery of your ailment. You have every reason to expect that they will succeed—perhaps in time to help you, for the pace of scientific advance grows faster every year. This is largely because research today is increasingly a team effort. The lone scientific explorer, like Pasteur who discovered by himself that germs cause infection, is of a bygone age.

Today, by publishing reports of their investigations and results and by reading what others have done, scientists keep in touch with one another's efforts. That saves them from duplicating mistakes and unnecessary trial and error; it makes it possible for each investigator to draw on the observations of others in interpreting his own results. Just as a runner in a relay race, one scientist takes up the work where the other leaves off.

The American Heart Association, an institution to which you owe more than you perhaps realize, is an active agent in collecting funds for financing the research in this area. The Association's contribution to hastening the day of enlightenment is enormous. Thousands of hypertensive patients—you may be one of them—are alive today because of knowledge gleaned from research financed by it. The American Heart Association, as well as all legitimate research centers and organizations that help in its financing, deserves your generous support.

Remember that in the last few years we have seen pneumonia and other forms of infection, including infections of the heart (until then, formidable agents of death), robbed of their terrors by penicillin and other antibiotics. We have seen the conquest of malaria, which for centuries scourged widespread populations. Perhaps finest of all, we are reaping the benefits of vaccines and modern sanitation in preventing yellow fever, smallpox, typhoid fever, and a host of other mass killers which periodically swept over large parts of the world in epidemic forms.

Now we await medication that will end high blood pressure. As you know, we already have some effective medications for control, brought about by researchers. I have tried in this book to tell you of the latest ideas among medical scientists for living safely and comfortably with high blood pressure. If you take an intelligent attitude toward your disorder, live according to the rules, keep in regular touch with your doctor and follow his advice, you should enjoy a satisfactory life—I hope a long life, long enough perhaps to see the complete conquest of high blood pressure.

Appendix I

DESIRABLE WEIGHT FOR MEN
Courtesy Metropolitan Life Insurance Company

HEIGHT
(with shoes on—
1-inch heels)

Weight in Pounds According to Frame
(as ordinarily dressed)

feet	inches	small frame	medium frame	large frame
5	2	116-125	124-133	131-142
5	3	119-128	127-136	133-144
5	4	122-132	130-140	137-149
5	5	126-136	134-144	141-153
5	6	129-139	137-147	145-157
5	7	133-143	141-151	149-162
5	8	136-147	145-156	153-166
5	9	140-151	149-160	157-170
5	10	144-155	153-164	161-175
5	11	148-159	157-168	165-180
6	0	152-164	161-173	169-185
6	1	157-169	166-178	174-190
6	2	163-175	171-184	179-196
6	3	168-180	176-189	184-202

DESIRABLE WEIGHT FOR WOMEN
Courtesy Metropolitan Life Insurance Company

HEIGHT
(with shoes on—
2-inch heels)

Weight in Pounds According to Frame
(as ordinarily dressed)

feet	inches	small frame	medium frame	large frame
4	11	104-111	110-118	117-127
5	0	105-113	112-120	119-129
5	1	107-115	114-122	121-131
5	2	110-118	117-125	124-135
5	3	113-121	120-128	127-138
5	4	116-125	124-132	131-142
5	5	119-128	127-135	133-145
5	6	123-132	130-140	138-150
5	7	126-136	134-144	142-154
5	8	129-139	137-147	145-158
5	9	133-143	141-151	149-162
5	10	136-147	145-155	152-166
5	11	139-150	148-158	155-169

For girls between 18 and 25, subtract 1 pound for each year under 25.

Appendix II
Diets Courtesy Dietetic Department, Michael Reese Hospital

DIET NUMBER 1

Furnishes about 1000 calories

Fat-free meat-stock soups	*As desired*
Lean meat, fish, poultry and cheese Omit pork and pork products Omit fried meats, fish and poultry Omit gravies	*2 small servings* *(2 oz. each)*
Eggs, any way except fried	*One*
Milk, Skim, or fat-free buttermilk	*1 pint*
Citrus fruits or tomatoes	*1 serving*
Fruits, fresh, or canned without sugar No dried fruit, banana, or avocado	*2 servings*
Green or yellow vegetables	*1-2 servings*
Other vegetables except potatoes, dried beans and peas, corn	*1-2 servings*
Bread: 1 serving of potatoes may substitute for 1 slice bread	*3 slices*
Desserts	*None except fruit as listed above*

Appendix II

Fats—butter or margarine — *1 pat. No other fat allowed as such or in cooking*

Sweets — *None. Saccharine may be used for sweetening*

Seasonings—salt, pepper, vinegar, spices, herbs — *As desired*

Beverages—tea, coffee; no sugar or cream — *As desired*

SUGGESTED MEAL PATTERN

Breakfast

Fruit or
Egg—one
Toast—1 slice
Butter—1 pat
Skim Milk—½ pint
Beverage—as indicated above

Dinner & Supper

Lean Meat—2 oz. serving
Cooked vegetable—1 serving
Raw vegetable salad—1 serving with lemon wedge or vinegar
Bread—1 slice
Fruit as indicated above— 1 serving
Beverage as specified or ½ pt. skim milk at one of these meals or at bedtime

DIET NUMBER 2

Furnishes about 1500 calories

Fat-free meat stock soups	As desired
Meat, fish, poultry and cheese Omit fried meats, fish and poultry Omit gravies	2 servings (2½ oz. each)
Eggs, any way except fried	One
Milk or Buttermilk	1 pint
Citrus fruits or tomatoes	1 serving
Fruits, fresh or canned without sugar No dried fruit, banana or avocado	2 servings
Green or yellow vegetables	1-2 servings
Other vegetables except potatoes, dried beans and peas, corn	1-2 servings
Bread: one serving of potato or one serving of cereal may be substituted for 1 slice bread	4 slices
Desserts	None except fruits listed above
Fats—butter or margarine	5 pats may be used as such or in cooking. 1 tablespoon cream may be substituted for 1 pat butter
Sweets	None. Saccharine may be used for sweetening
Seasonings—salt, pepper, vinegar, spices, herbs	As desired
Beverages—tea, coffee; no cream or sugar	As desired

SUGGESTED MEAL PATTERN

Breakfast

Fruit or fruit juice—1 serving
Egg—one
Toast—2 slices
Butter—2 pats
Beverage—as indicated above
Cream—1 Tbsp
Milk—½ pint

Dinner & Supper

Meat or substitute—2½ oz. serving
Cooked vegetable—1 serving
Raw vegetable salad—1 serving, with lemon wedge or vinegar
Bread—1 slice
Butter—1 pat
Fruit as indicated above—1 serving
½ pt. milk at one of these meals or bedtime

Appendix III

AGENCIES OF REHABILITATION AND VOCATIONAL PLACEMENT

The American Heart Association whose main office is located at 44 E. 23rd Street, New York 10, N.Y. is always ready to help and advise patients with disease of the heart and blood vessels. It also has affiliated societies in the larger cities of the United States which may be found in the local telephone directories.

These associations are voluntary health agencies devoted to combating premature death and disability from diseases of the heart and blood vessels. The members are private citizens, including physicians and others in many walks of life who have dedicated themselves to this work.

Resources and financial aid are given voluntarily by the general public. On the annual Tag Day the public is asked to donate to the Heart Fund. The slogan on the tag, "Have a Heart," means just what it says. The principal source of funds is the annual Heart Fund campaign. Other important financial contributions come through legacies, bequests and memorial gifts.

The money is used to gather useful information, to

sponsor research, to organize scientific meetings where physicians and other scientists may exchange new information, to educate the public in matters relating to diseases of the heart and blood vessels including high blood pressure and to further the rehabilitation of patients so that they can again become useful self-supporting citizens.

This is a great and worthy undertaking, open to all and deserving of your financial and moral support. In contributing to it, you are both helping science to broaden and increase our knowledge of one of man's greatest enemies, and contributing to the health and welfare of thousands of deserving men, women and children.

Other Agencies: Public

As a taxpayer, you have a right to draw upon the public agencies listed below. Do not hesitate to do so: you have paid for it in your taxes.

1. *Division of Vocational Rehabilitation or Education*

The State-Federal program of vocational rehabilitation operates in all forty-eight states. It is an important resource for placement of patients and any individual of working age is eligible to receive the benefits of its services. The agency offers the following services:

Rehabilitation diagnosis and evaluation of the kind of work the patient might do.

Provision of medical services when necessary.

Vocational training in school, on the job, or in sheltered workshops.

Financial support for various purposes when necessary.

Vocational guidance, counseling, placement and follow-up.

There is no charge for these services. Application can be made by the physician or the patient himself to the Division of Vocational Rehabilitation which is usually located in the capital city of the state and listed in the telephone directory under State Department of Education. There are branch offices in the principal cities in some states.

2. *State Employment Service*

In every state the State Employment Service, usually a subdivision of the Division of Placement and Unemployment Insurance, State Department of Labor, operates a service for the handicapped. Guidance and placement services are rendered without cost to the applicant. It is advisable that the physician mail a written report on the physical condition of the applicant together with an appraisal of the type of work which is suitable for the particular patient. The State Employment Office is usually listed in the telephone directory under State Department of Labor.

3. *Veterans Administration*

Veterans may receive assistance from the local Veterans Hospital or Veterans Administration office in the form of guidance, placement and sometimes vocational training.

4. *Old Age Assistance*

Patients over sixty-five years of age may call and make use of the Bureau of Old Age Assistance which is generally under the auspices of the Department of Welfare of the city or county.

There are other agencies, some of them operating for a fee, that can help in placement and rehabilitation. The local heart association or the local health department can usually provide information concerning the location of such agencies in the community.

Private Agencies

1. *National Society for Crippled Children and Adults*

This society is active in all forty-eight states and is usually located in the capital city of the state and is listed in the telephone directory under the name of the state. It offers vocational counseling, training and placement services in some instances, but will always supply the physician with information concerning the availability of such services in the community.

2. *Sheltered Workshops and Rehabilitation Institutes*

Several sheltered workshops, such as Goodwill Industries, are national in scope. Other rehabilitation centers are frequently connected with universities, medical schools, hospitals and welfare centers. Many sheltered workshops will employ patients who, because of age or partial disability cannot find work in the open labor market.

3. *Industry*

When a patient returns to his former job, or to one in the same industry which is less taxing, his physician should communicate with the medical service department at the plant. This will frequently facilitate return to suitable work in an appropriate occupation.

Index

Abdominal (Peritoneal) Dialysis, 119
Aches and pains, as symptoms of hypertension, 27
Adrenal glands, 123–124
Age, and susceptibility to hypertension, 36–38, 41, 56
Albumin, 70–71
American Heart Association, 131
Amphetamines, 87–88
Angina Pectoris, 99–100
Antihypertensives, 52–54
Antiotonin, 110
Aorta, 13, 15, 19, 21, 65, 97
    coarctation of, 107–109
Appetite suppressants, 87–88
Arteries, 25, 65, 73–74, 76, 94–97
    coronary, 98
    function of, 18–19
    strength of, 5–6
Arterioles, 18, 19, 97
Arteriosclerosis, 2, 25, 41, 50, 94–97, 98, 101
Artificial kidney, 113–119

Blacks, incidence of hypertension among, 38–39, 51
Blood circulation, 18–22, 97
Blood pressure
    daily changes in, 9–10
    maximum, 42–43
    measurement of, 64–70
    normal, 14–15
Body build, and susceptibility to hypertension, 42
Breathing, examination of, 60
Bright, Richard, 71
Bright's disease. *See* Nephritis

Capillaries, 19–20
Casts, 71
Chest, examination of, 62–63
Chinese, incidence of hypertension among, 38
Chlorthiazide, 53
Cholesterol, 94
Circulatory system, 18–22, 97
Coarctation of the aorta, 107–109
Collateral circulation, 101–103
Coronary thrombosis, 100
Cortisone, 124
Crossness, as symptom of hypertension, 29
Cushing, Dr. Harvey W., 123–124
Cushing's syndrome, 123–124

Dexedrine, 87–88
Diagnosis by a physician, 29–33, 44–46, 125–126
Dialysis, 113–119
Diastolic pressure, 15, 23, 50
    measurement of, 68–70
Dieting to lose weight, 86–91
Differential diagnosis, 45–46
Dizziness, as symptom of hypertension, 27–28, 60
Doctors
    examination by, 56–74
    importance of, 44–46, 125

Emotional symptoms of hypertension, 28, 35–36, 58–59
Epinephrine, 121
Essential hypertension, 13–14, 23, 34, 75
    complications of, 94–106

Essential hypertension (*cont.*)
  symptoms of, 23–29
  treatment of, 52–55
Examination by a physician, 56–74
Exercise, 92
Eyes, examination of, 72–74

Fat-free diets, 89
Fatigue, as symptom of hypertension, 28–29
Fear accompanying hypertension, 5, 99, 105–106
Food fads, 88–89
Framingham study of hypertensives, 49–51
"Frozen Woman" of Chicago, 9–10

Goldblatt, Dr. Harry, 109–110

Hales, Stephen, 65
Headaches
  as symptom of hypertension, 24–27
  warnings on, 25–27
Heart
  complications of, 97–100
  enlargement of, 98
  examination of, 63–64
  function of, 18–19, 20–21
Heredity
  and obesity, 85
  and susceptibility to hypertension, 30, 34–35, 57
High blood pressure. *See* Hypertension
Hydralazine, 54–55
Hypertension
  early treatment of, 2, 50–51
  and heredity, 30, 34–35
  and modern civilization, 8–9, 41–42
  recent findings concerning, 1–6
  recovery from, 106
  treatment of, 47–55
  types of, 23
  See also Essential hypertension Secondary hypertension
Hypertensive people
  how to help oneself, 76–93
  rules to follow, 125–129
Hypotension, 10–12
  postural, 11–12
  primary (essential), 10–11
  secondary, 11

Inferior vena cava, 20
Insomnia, as symptom of hypertension, 28–29
Intima, 94
Intravenous pyelogram, 111

Jews, incidence of hypertension among, 39

Kidney ailments
  diagnosis of, 70–72
  recent treatment of, 1–2, 113–121
  See also Nephritis, Uremia
Kidney transplants, 119–121
Kidneys, efficiency of, 71–72
Korotkow, 66, 68

Left auricle of heart, 20–21
Left ventricle of heart, 19
Low blood pressure. *See* Hypotension
Lungs, 63
Lymphocytes, 120

Menopause, 36–37
Michigan Heart Association, 39
Milk farms, 90–91
Modern civilization, 8–9, 41–42

INDEX

Nephritis (Bright's disease), 71, 109–110, 111
Nitroglycerine, 100
Norepinephrine, 121

Obesity, 80–84
  how to avoid, 84–93
  and hypertension, 16–17, 42
Obstructive strokes, 101–104

Paralysis, as a result of a stroke, 103–104
Pharmaceuticals used in treating hypertension, 51–55
Pheochromocytoma, 121–122
Physical examination by a physician, 59–66
Pill, contraceptive, 124
Postural hypotension, 11–12
Potassium, loss of, 123
Pregnancy, 80
Primary hyperaldosteronism, 122–123
Primary hypotension, 10–11
Pulse, 61–62
Pyelogram, 72

Race, and incidence of hypertension, 9, 38–40, 51
Renal function tests, 72
Reserpine, 54
Rest, importance of, 76–78, 126
Right auricle of heart, 20
Right ventricle of heart, 20
Riva-Rocci, 65–66

Salt-free diets, 89, 112–113
Secondary hypertension, 13, 23, 52, 59–60
  ailments causing, 107–124

Secondary hypotension, 11
Sex, and susceptibility to hypertension, 36–37
Sexual abstinence, 79
Smoking, 58, 89–90
Spas, 78–79
Sphygmomanometer, 64–70
Spinal test, 104
Starzl, Dr., 120
Steam baths, 93
Stethoscope, 64
Stroke caused by bleeding, 104–105
Strokes, 100–105
Superior vena cava, 20
Surgical reduction of weight, 91–92
Systolic pressure, 15, 50
  measurement of, 66–68

Temperament, and susceptibility to hypertension, 35–36
Thiazides, 52–54
Thyroid, 87

Uremia, 110–112
Urine tests, 70–72

Veins, 20
Vertigo, 27
Veterans' Administration report on treatment of hypertension, 51

Weight control, 127
Weight reduction, 84–93
Work for hypertensives, 127
Worry, danger of, 128